Changing
Normal

Changing Normal

How I Helped My Husband Beat Cancer

MARILU HENNER
and MICHAEL BROWN

Gallery Books

NEW YORK LONDON TORONTO SYDNEY NEW DELHI

G

Gallery Books
An Imprint of Simon & Schuster, Inc.
1230 Avenue of the Americas
New York, NY 10020

First Gallery Books hardcover edition April 2016

GALLERY BOOKS and colophon are registered
trademarks of Simon & Schuster, Inc.

For information about special discounts for bulk purchases,
please contact Simon & Schuster Special Sales at
1-866-506-1949 or business@simonandschuster.com.

The Simon & Schuster Speakers Bureau can bring authors to your live event. For
more information or to book an event, contact the Simon & Schuster Speakers
Bureau at 1-866-248-3049 or visit our website at www.simonspeakers.com.

Interior design by Renato Stanisic

Manufactured in the United States of America

10 9 8 7 6 5 4 3 2 1

Library of Congress Cataloging-in-Publication Data is available.

ISBN 978-1-4767-9394-8
ISBN 978-1-4767-9395-5 (ebook)

MARILU

To Michael:
For his love and trust, and, most of all, for his ability
to seek the truth and do something about it.

And to my parents, Joe and Loretta:
Whose lives and deaths inspire me every day
to find a healthier way to live and to share
what I learn with anyone who will listen.

MICHAEL

I want to dedicate this book to my parents, Bill
and LaRae, who did their best with their
wayward son. And to Marilu, without whom this
story would not have happened, nor been told.

first met Mike Brown in 2003 when my longtime and dear patient Marilu Henner first brought him into my practice in Los Angeles and explained that he was her new boyfriend. Although Michael is a big, strapping man, he looked pale, worn out, depleted, and his body language told me that he was sad and dejected.

With Marilu in the room, I asked Mike to describe his health issues and reasons for seeing me, an integrative medicine doctor. He explained that he had been diagnosed with bladder cancer. I was shocked to learn that he had been symptomatic for two years, and yet, despite consulting with a specialist during this time, had never been properly diagnosed.

A patient's body language and speech are as important as his clinical diagnosis, and Mike's body language was saying, *I am a sick man.*

As an integrative medicine doctor, I recognize that health is on a spectrum. At one end of the scale, we have optimal well-being, and, at the other end, degenerative disease. What we are not taught in medical school, even to this day, is that there is a gray zone in the middle. In this zone, organ dysfunction is occurring long before any clinical disease is diagnosed. These dysfunctions must be treated, whether they're caused by cancer, diabetes, chronic fatigue, or any other chronic disease. Integrative doctors are able to address these dysfunctions to bring organs back into normal function.

The imbalances and dysfunctions of organs—without frank, identifiable disease—occur for years before the disease is recognized. This is why cancer is so hard to cure. For example, cancer kinetics tell us that a one-centimeter lump in a woman with breast cancer means that the cancer has been growing for about four years. That's four years lost without a remedy.

In Michael's case, because he had been diagnosed with bladder cancer, it was very important we address his history with toxic exposures because bladder cancer is typically associated with toxic environmental exposures. Michael's personal history, as he outlines in this book, was overwhelmed by toxic exposures. From the cigarettes he smoked to all the toxins on the ships he worked on, including solvents, PCBs, phthalates, pesticides, and heavy metals, he unfortunately became a perfect candidate to develop bladder cancer.

Over the course of the ensuing months, while he was receiving traditional treatment for his bladder cancer, Michael and I looked at his blood and urine tests showing the degree of toxins he had been exposed to in his life.

All of us are exposed to some toxicity in our lives, which is called our *exposome*. The lifetime accumulation of a patient's exposome is called *total body burden*. When total body burden exceeds a patient's genetics and organ toleration, he will develop either inflammatory or degenerative conditions. In Michael's case, he developed cancer.

In addition, because 50 to 80 percent of our immune system is in our gut, it was very important to look at Michael's intestinal function. Over our months together, we continued to address issues such as intestinal permeability problems and dysbiosis, which developed due to his diet and lifestyle.

We also looked at his stress system. Many years ago, I routinely talked to patients with chronic illness about the role that stress played. This was considered radical by colleagues. Now, however, major universities have departments of psychoneuroimmunology that study the role that stress plays on our immune system and how that affects our health.

When I looked at Michael's stress system, through both saliva hormone tests and acupuncture meridian testing, I found his immune system and nutrient levels to be completely depleted by the years of stress he endured before his diagnosis. With herbal therapy, acupuncture treatments, nutritional supplements, and major changes in his diet, over the ensuing months, his stress system gradually became more balanced. Fortunately, Michael's girlfriend—and now wife—was Marilu! Her knowledge of the role of diet, as well as her ability to prepare wholesome food for him and get him off junk food, were huge factors in turning around his health.

When the subsequent diagnosis of lung cancer came along, we were already supporting Michael's entire system. Michael was already into his new lifestyle. His immune tests, stress tests, and toxicity levels continued to improve.

Over our years together, not only cleaning out his toxins and changing his diet but also the transformation of his lifestyle allowed him to remain perfectly healthy in spite of his two diagnoses of cancer. Michael was a very diligent patient who was willing to try anything to help his body heal. A good patient is one who takes responsibility for their own care and who seeks to understand what they can do to aid the doctor in realizing their own recovery. Without his own determination to be saved, nothing that Marilu and I did would have been enough to save Michael.

The most recent medical literature has shown that up to 80 percent of our health is determined by our lifestyle.

The title of Marilu and Michael's book, *Changing Normal*, could not be more reflective of the transition Michael has gone through, which has allowed him to reclaim his health. Michael has gone from a stressed-out, toxic, dejected, junk-food-eating person with a diagnosis of cancer to his current "new" self—a man with a strong immune system and a balanced stress system, a healthy eater, and a positive thinker.

So much of conventional cancer therapy is focused on killing the cancer, while *integrative* medicine offers support to the immune, endocrine, digestive, and nervous systems as another way to make sure cancer does not return.

We each need to look at what we have been defining as "normal." In our current society in America, it is normal to eat fast foods, not exercise, be constantly stressed, and remain overweight most of our lives. And then, in our thirties and forties, it is normal to start using pharmaceuticals to control—but not cure—the diseases we get: high blood pressure, diabetes, heart disease, cancer, and others.

Just by changing our definition of normal to a diet that is clean, with wholesome, fresh organic foods, and a lifestyle of regular exercise and activities and hobbies that keep us happy, we can change the healthcare system of America to one that is wellness-focused, rather than disease-fixing.

It is up to all of us to bring this transformation to our own lives as Michael did to his.

Soram Khalsa, MD
December 2015

Changing
Normal

This Is Your Lucky Day!

Think of your body as a field of soil. If a weed sprouts up, it's not enough to cut out that weed and then poison the soil. You have to change the soil, fertilize it with different nutrients, and lovingly tend to it for another weed not to grow.

Marilu

I had to remember to breathe. Exhale deliberately so that I could inhale enough breath to look calm.

Michael and I rode the elevator in silence except for a knowing smile between us when an older, still affectionate couple got on; a spontaneous kiss when they exited on their floor. All it took was a look into each other's eyes to know that no matter what was ahead for us, we'd be okay. Michael and I had known each other for decades, but we'd only been dating three months. Already we knew we were in it for keeps.

I took another deep breath and the elevator door opened. The receptionist noted Michael's name and led us to a waiting room. We picked our seats, and, for the third time that week, Michael filled in a set of papers explaining why he was seeing a doctor.

He had bladder cancer.

After having blood in his urine (hematuria) for more than two years, Michael had finally been diagnosed. But not by his urologist, who saw him several times and sent him home chalking it up to possible kidney stones, gall stones, even the ridiculous notion of his having taken too many supplements—something I'd never heard of in all my years of studying health. That doctor never tested any further, no matter how much blood there was or how often the hematuria occurred. This was unacceptable in my book. So now Michael was counting on me because of my advocacy and connections to the health community. I did my due diligence and found one of the top bladder cancer specialists in America, and, lucky for us, he happened to be in Los Angeles. We made the appointment looking for answers to questions we didn't yet know to ask.

Michael

In contemporary America, it is neither polite nor politically correct to talk about what might have been in cancer treatments; one must not ask the patient if they regret the surgery, the radiation, the chemo. That is rude, bad taste. These people have been brave, taken their medicine, fought the good fight; to now ask hard questions, to cast doubt on their actions, seems to be pointless nitpicking. Didn't they do everything that could be done? Not only that, aren't they only asking for the right to return to normal, to have a few more months or years to live the way they used to, the way that possibly got them the cancer in the first place?

Marilu

While Michael filled in the paperwork, I picked up an issue of *People* magazine, trying to distract myself with "The World's Most Beautiful People" as much as I was trying to ground myself for what could come next. For years, I've been known among my friends as the "Doctor Concierge," a collector of MDs of all stripes ever since I started to study and write about health. After my mother's death from the complications of rheumatoid arthritis in 1978, I have had an interest in connecting people to the right health and medical information. She was only fifty-eight years old, and when she died, I vowed to learn everything I could about the human body and to share the information with anyone who would listen. Thus far this knowledge has allowed me to help many people with arthritis and cardiovascular disease—which killed my father when he was only fifty-two—as well as people who struggled with their weight and skin issues, just as I had for so many years before finding a better way to eat and live.

But I had never taken on the task of helping someone who had cancer. And here I was, with the love of my life, someone I had known since we were eighteen and freshmen at the University of Chicago, both of us then living richly textured lives with big careers, three marriages, and five kids between us, and then reuniting two months prior to his fateful diagnosis.

Could what I had learned from my decades of seeing life through the prism of health help Michael put his cancer in remission? Could the same principles used in reversing cardiovascular disease and ameliorating the symptoms of arthritis and Crohn's disease be applied to something as complex as cancer? Could the diet I've been following for more than thirty years—writing nine books celebrating its healthy effects on my weight and well-being—actually help save Michael's life and "cure" his cancer?

And maybe the biggest question of all—Was I in over my head?

Michael

When a person gets sick with cancer, the questions *why me*, *why this cancer*, and *what could I have done* are constant companions. After my diagnosis, I lay in bed at night wondering what chemical, what pollutant inspired my tumors to grow like they did. Looking deeper, I saw the toxic waste dump deep in my cells—my body was polluted, and I was living in an acidic sea that was nurturing my bladder cancer. Doctors tell us patients that we will never know why we got the cancer. Genetics? Maybe. Environment, lifestyle, stress? All of these are factors, and the doctor will agree. But he will not urge the patient to go deeper. To do so would be akin to blaming the patient for his disease. Rather than using the natural curiosity of the patient as a way to search for the cause of the cancer so that it can be addressed, the patient is given homilies about how the cancer was random, unusual, unique even. Meanwhile, all of these unusual and unique cancers are subject to the same radical therapies: surgery, radiation, and chemo.

Marilu

As Michael's personal Doctor Concierge I knew I wanted him to visit every great doctor I've known over the years to see if we could put together the best protocol for him to follow. But we were only together two months when he was diagnosed, and I had no idea how committed he would be to the alternative methods I so strongly believed in. In my mind, it would be a combination of Eastern and Western medicine—the best of both worlds—because, by this time in my health journey, I had worked with the greatest doctors of integrative medicine in the country. These doctors analyze everything about a patient—body, mind, and spirit. And they look at the body as a whole, not just one part at a time. They combine complementary and alternative medicine (acupuncture, osteopathy, chiropractic, massage, supplementation, meditation, ayurvedic medicine, and so on) with the more science-based healthcare practices. I knew that—in addition to whatever any doctor recommended—diet, exercise, and major detox would have to be at the base of Michael's healing.

I assumed we would also consult the more typical AMA (American Medical Association) doctors, who might advise him to take the more conventional routes the world has come to know as cancer patient care. When hearing Michael had cancer, people were quick to tell us their stories of chemo and radiation, whether it be their own treatment or that of someone they knew. But only the people in the holistic health world talked about reversing their cancers through a vegan or macrobiotic diet, visualization, supplements, chelation, skin brushing, colon therapy, and so on.

Michael and I were going to leave no stone unturned. I felt responsible for presenting him with every option available. We would hear what everyone had to say, listen to what made the most sense, and then, hopefully, use our judgment as to what to put into action, together.

Michael

Doctors believe in their treatments, they are invested in that world. For most of them, alternative treatments are totally alien or not really treatments at all. They may be as good as lifestyle changes, but they are not effective in treating disease. This goes beyond cancer to include all sorts of maladies. High blood pressure is treated with pills, not changes in diet. And so are cholesterol, constipation, and colitis. The focus is always the disease rather than the patient. The disease is treated, not the organism, not the body as a whole. But if the entire body is not treated, not brought into balance, then the cancer will almost invariably return, despite the best efforts of conventional medicine.

Marilu

The doctor's assistant, much like the maître d' in a restaurant, came out into the waiting room to greet the next set of patients and recognized me instantly. To be honest, I was thinking, *Thank God* for *Taxi*! There's nothing like a little extra help when you're fighting for a life. The assistant introduced himself and looked over Michael's chart, which had been sent ahead of our visit, and seemed to know what was coming for us. With a big smile on his face he said, "This is your lucky day!"

Michael asked, "It is? Why?"

"Because there's a cancellation on Wednesday!" He beamed. "This is your lucky day. The doctor will explain."

He led us into an office, not an examination room, and told us the doctor would be with us soon.

Staring at us around the office were the various diplomas, awards, and credentials of this well-known bladder cancer surgeon, which made us feel confident that Michael's condition would be a been-there, done-that situation for him. I smiled at Michael and grabbed his hand, hopefully reassuringly. The actor in me wanted to pretend I wasn't scared, but I was. Shortly thereafter the distinguished-looking, white-haired, no-nonsense doctor breezed into the room with his adoring assistant in tow and shook our hands. Barely glancing at Michael's chart, he set to work, pulling out a piece of blank paper and beginning to sketch out his plans.

As if we were on the same team in Pictionary, he drew illustrations of Michael's inner organs, saying, "I have a cancellation on Wednesday. I'm going to take out the bladder. I'm going to take out the prostate, too, because that's how the surgery is done. And then I'm going to pull down a piece of your intestine to make a neobladder." The assistant told us that this was a technique for which the doctor was famous. The doctor continued by explaining, "I'm going to place it right behind your navel, which is the best place to put it."

Michael and I were aghast. We sat there in silence long enough for the doctor to notice. Based on our horrified expressions, he tried to reassure us: "And don't worry if the two of you want to have sex. I'm going to run a small inflatable hose up your penis, and every time you want to make love, you just have to pump it up six times."

"Well, can we have the seven-pump model?" I felt compelled to inquire. " 'Cause we're a sexy couple!"

The doctor laughed as the assistant said, "Tell them about the sheik!"

In graphic detail, the doctor described how a sheik had come to see him when the sheik had been diagnosed with bladder cancer, since he had heard that this doctor was the best in the world at this procedure. He had asked the doctor to assure him that after the surgery he would still be man enough to satisfy his four wives. "No problem!" the great doctor had told him. Besides pioneering the neobladder, this surgeon had also developed a pump technique that could not only preserve a man's sexual prowess after losing his bladder and prostate, but, in many cases, actually improve it. The sheik, in fact, had come back to proclaim that, indeed, it was true that his sexual prowess had remained strong, and that he was considering taking another wife into his harem, so satisfied were his wives and him with his lovemaking ability!

The bladder?

The prostate?

A pump?

Six- or seven-pump model, I didn't care. The blood was rushing to my head, but I had to ask, "And what about nutrition and health? Anything Michael should do, or eat, or not eat for his bladder cancer?"

He looked at Michael and said, "Nah," chuckling at the absurdity of my question. "Have all the steak and highballs you want."

Michael

Each patient, if they survive their conventional cancer treatment, then becomes an advocate for that treatment. Of course, if they are unwilling to question their actions or reflect on their treatment and its consequences, then they must believe it was the correct treatment. If they begin to doubt the wisdom of their doctors, then their caregivers also feel like they have failed. The caregivers have a stake in this, too; they are the ones who agreed to the procedures, who urged the patient to take his or her medicine. A conspiracy of silence is created that results in others getting the same treatment. How many men must regret the prostate surgery that left them impotent while suffering the pain and discomfort they will endure the rest of their lives? How many women have had both breasts removed because of an early-stage tumor that may or may not have resulted in full-blown breast cancer? The need for radical action in the face of cancer, aside from those diagnosed with advanced stage 4, stems from the doctor's belief that the patient will never change and it is his job to return the patient to normal. If this were not true, then watchful waiting combined with lifestyle changes would be the norm, rather than the exception. But patients, so out of touch with their bodies, are made to believe that cutting out the tumor will cure the cancer, when it does nothing of the kind.

Marilu

We said our goodbyes to the doctor and told him we'd call him later that day to let him know about surgery next Wednesday.

We rode the elevator down in silence, not knowing what to say, even to each other. The option presented by the doctor was so far beyond what we expected to hear that both of us were processing the information as best we could. The Rolodex in my brain was flipping through other doctors' names and anything else I could think of when it came to cancer. It all just sounded so extreme. There had to be another way.

Michael broke the silence when we reached our car, turning to me, saying, "They're not cutting into me. I'm not losing my bladder."

"Okay," I said. "We'll look at all the alternatives. We'll see the doctors I know. We'll figure it out."

Michael nodded in agreement.

I reassured him, "And no matter what, we're in this together." And I started to say what I was really thinking—*I didn't finally connect with the love of my life to carve him up or have him die*—but at that point, Michael didn't need to hear anything more about his possible future. It was time to go to work.

OVER THE PAGES OF THIS book, Michael and I will tell our stories, individually and as a couple. You will read about my health and weight struggles and how I lowered my cholesterol over one hundred points, permanently lost fifty-four pounds, and changed my entire lifestyle after my parents' deaths inspired me to become a student of health. And you will come to understand how Michael's quest to become a man in the adventure-seeking, drinking, smoking, and womanizing ways of the world led to his lifetime accumulation of bad habits and toxic exposures. Michael and I will tell our story of meeting as freshmen at the University of Chicago, running into each other in New Orleans days before I married my first husband, falling in love after not seeing each other for more than twenty-two years only to discover, within months, that he had not one, but two cancers—bladder and lung—and we will share what he did to put his cancer in remission for more than twelve years now. It is not only *our* love story, it is the story of how the *human body* loves to survive and thrive and heal itself, as long as you do right by it. And it is the story of strengthening the immune system, saving organs, and eschewing chemo and radiation—a story of love, detox, and changing normal.

And, just for the record, no pump necessary.

If you go to a doctor and all he says is, "Let's cut out that cancer and then give you chemo and radiation. You'll be back to normal in no time." Please run far away from anyone who wants you to go back to normal. Normal is probably what got you into trouble in the first place. Normal has to be looked at. Normal has to be changed.

CHAPTER ONE

Marilu

I grew up in Logan Square on the Northwest Side of Chicago in a typical two-flat, but our family was anything but typical. My mother's love of dance prompted our father to turn our garage into a dance studio so that she and five of her six kids could teach dancing to two hundred students between the ages of two and eighty, including the nuns from the Catholic church next door who came over for stretch classes. Each week the students showed up to learn ballet, tap, jazz, ballroom, and social dancing. The Friday night teenage classes were particularly popular, with raging hormones and wafting pheromones. I'm sure that most kids in my neighborhood had their first kiss somewhere on our property.

Everyone loved my parents. My dad was the guy you called if you were in trouble; my mom was the mom you called when you had a problem. She always said that he was book smart and she was people smart. It was a winning combination. Because of the popularity of the dancing school, we were the epicenter of the neighborhood and thought of ourselves as the Kennedys of Logan Square. But the dancing school wasn't enough for my mom. She also ran a beauty shop out of our kitchen, where twenty-five women from the neighborhood would come for cuts, perms, and dye jobs. The kitchen was set up like a hair salon to the point that the refrigerator was on the stairway to the basement, and in its place sat a blue hair-drying chair straight out of *Steel Magnolias*.

Besides having a dancing school in our garage and a beauty shop in our kitchen, my mother's brother, our uncle, lived upstairs with ten cats, two dogs, two birds, a skunk, 150 fish, and his boyfriend, Charles. "Uncle," as everyone in the neighborhood called him, also taught art at the Catholic grammar school next door and held art classes after school while the dancing school and beauty shop were in full swing. He was also the neighborhood astrologist and ran a cat hospital on our roof in a structure that was once a small homemade greenhouse.

Needless to say, my family life was very special and different, and my parents' and uncle's creative and entrepreneurial spirits were an integral part of my growing up that continues to inform my life to this day. The Henner house was not only colorful and somewhat eccentric—with six very smart siblings vying for space and time—but it was also academic and highly competitive, thanks to our father's intelligence and salesmanship. I was also born with an unusual memory—now called HSAM for Highly Superior Autobiographical Memory—that makes it possible for me to remember every day of my life and everything that ever happens to me. So it was never a question of whether or not I would go to college; it was only a question of where.

I FIRST FELL IN LOVE with the University of Chicago on Sunday October 6, 1968, when, as a Madonna High School junior from

Chicago's Northwest Side, I represented my school at a communications event. As soon as I walked on the campus, saw the ivy-covered Gothic buildings, and felt the gravitas of the university's rich intellectual history, I knew this would be my college. It may have been my first visit to U of C, but the school already held a special place in my heart due to the fact that my father had gone there for a six-week course after serving in the Air Force during World War II.

Being a good student with four scholarships to prove it—including having been named Outstanding Teenager of Illinois—I knew I could probably get into any college upon which I set my sights. But because I also had this burning desire to be an actress—as a teenager I had always been performing in a play somewhere in the city—my choices upon graduation were either to go straight to New York to become a professional actress or to go to the best school in Chicago and continue taking advantage of my community theater contacts. But after my father passed away during Christmas break of my senior year in high school, I knew there wasn't really a question. I was definitely going to apply to the University of Chicago and stay in my hometown. When the large acceptance packet arrived on Wednesday, April 15, 1970, I felt that my father had arranged it from afar.

My father's death and the way he died—a heart attack during an argument with one of my brothers at our dancing school Christmas party—was such a shock to all of us that I found myself eating my feelings and putting on a lot of weight, especially during the summer between high school and college. In September 1970, I started my freshman year at the University of Chicago with my weight at an all-time high. I was not anywhere near feeling *my best* and would catch myself constantly telling people, "This is not what I really look like."

Never one to feel sorry for myself, until I could get back to looking like the real me—which ended up taking several years—I decided to throw myself into being very colorful and theatrical from the *If you can't hide it, decorate it* school of life. I ran around campus during freshman orientation wearing an enormous figure-hiding black-and-rust-colored cape, which somehow, despite my insecurities, landed me on the cover of *Women's Wear Daily*. I guess big, dark, and oddball were in that year.

In 1970, the University of Chicago was unlike any other school in the country. My dorm, Woodward Court, was not only one of the first coed dorms in existence, its bathrooms were also coed. You could take a shower with your boyfriend or end up in a stall next to your crush from the down the hall—not my favorite thing about coed dorm life. I found it so uncomfortable, in fact, to use the bathroom next to guys that when my dorm held what they intended to be an anonymous ballot to determine whether or not they needed to make one of the four bathrooms women only, I raised my hand and said, "No need to make the ballots anonymous. You can put that non-coed bathroom right near my room." And they did. I can't tell you how many female dorm mates thanked me for what I didn't even consider a brave move. I'm a girl who loves options, and the idea that I could have my privacy in a stall *or* go down the hall to shower with my boyfriend in another bathroom seemed like the best of both worlds. I've never been one to back off from voicing my opinion, even when it's not the popular one.

The University of Chicago had several residential halls and, just like Hogwarts, each one seemed to house a different type of student. Woodward Court was located a block from the main part of campus, known as the Quadrangle, and it was divided by six houses: Upper and Lower Flint, Upper and Lower Rickert, and

Upper and Lower Wallace. Being the only coed dorm at U of C, with its sterile, modern rooms—cinder-block walls, casement windows, orange-and-green chenille bedspreads—it was inhabited, for the most part, by atypical University of Chicago students. In other words, the fun kids. The unofficial motto of the school at that time was "Where fun goes to die," but few of us living in Woodward Court acted like it. There was one pretty vivacious blonde named Linda with whom I hit it off immediately because she seemed like someone who would have been my friend no matter how we met. She and I bonded over our outgoing personalities, similar senses of humor, and definite boy craziness. When we first connected, she was very excited about having already met someone the first week of freshman orientation, and she was absolutely crazy about him. When our resident head and his wife invited Linda and me and four of our other dorm mates to a Friday night dinner, Linda arranged for her new boyfriend to pick her up so that we could all meet this mystery man.

I was feeling particularly vulnerable that night because of my weight but tried to hide it by pouring my then size 14 body into a size 12 dress that friends nicknamed the "bowling-ball dress" because of the way my cleavage looked. (I'm one of those people who get cleavage for free, just like Tina Fey. We also both have pointy eyeballs and can't wear contacts. It must be a Greek thing!) This dress was so Kardashian, long before there even was such a thing, that at the dinner the headmaster's slightly tipsy wife came after me waving their daughter's pull toy, screaming, "Homewrecker!" when her husband and I were just *talking*. I was shocked, embarrassed, and afraid of getting clocked by a Fisher-Price ball popper because nothing could have been further from the truth. I wasn't a homewrecker; I was just a self-conscious, overweight eighteen-year-old freshman girl wearing a too tight dress, trying to fit in. (Literally and figuratively!)

So imagine my relief when I could excuse myself to answer the doorbell.

And there he was.

Michael.

Tall, with shoulder-length hair and piercing blue eyes, and definitely the handsomest guy on campus. He filled the doorway and took my breath away. I adored Linda and, of course, didn't dare *twinkle* in Michael's direction, but I couldn't help but wonder, *If I lost the extra weight, would there be any more guys on campus like him?*

OVER THE NEXT FEW MONTHS I watched Linda and Michael's relationship grow from cute campus couple to raging sex maniacs. Once she walked the well-worn path from the freshman dorm to Billings Hospital to get birth control pills to lose her virginity to him, they hung a yellow ribbon around the door handle at all hours of the day and night to signal to her roommate, Kathi, and me to keep out! As a woman of experience who had lost my virginity the night of Neil Armstrong's moonwalk the year before, I was only too happy to give advice and share stories of my eighteen-year-old sexcapades. My neighborhood boyfriend, Steve, and I would often double-date with Linda and Michael. They even came to see me in an off-campus community theater production that took me away from school most weekends during the winter and spring quarters that year.

A former castmate of mine from Chicago community theater, Jim Jacobs, called me one day and said, "Henner! I've written this show. It may never get off the ground. We're going to perform it in a converted trolley barn on Lincoln Avenue called the Kingston Mine's Company Store. I wrote it about the kids I went to high school with, and even though you're younger, you've always reminded me of one of those girls." I showed up for the first read-through, and Jim handed each of us two stacks of papers nine inches high. One was a stack of music, and the other of scenes depicting high school life: the Book Report Scene, the Polio Shot Scene, the Lunchroom Scene, the Pajama Party Scene, the Rumble Scene, and so on. We workshopped the show for several weeks and on Friday February 5, 1971, ninety people saw the very first performance of *Grease*.

BESIDES OUR CONNECTION THROUGH LINDA, Michael and I also shared a required science core curriculum class every Tuesday and Thursday. For whatever reason, we had both chosen a physics class taught by Melba Phillips who, according to U of C legend, had been mistress to Enrico Fermi—the man who built the first nuclear reactor. (This was quite hard to believe, considering she looked nothing like a mistress and more like Eleanor Roosevelt's less attractive sister.) She was the only teacher in my entire school career who just plain hated me and told me I was too flamboyant for a college student. After our class, Michael and I would walk across campus together so that he could eat at our dorm cafeteria with Linda, because his no-frills dorm didn't have a meal plan. He and I would talk about the class and Linda and Chicago and our lives, but I held back from asking any really personal questions he would be reluctant to answer, as Michael is not one for idle chatter, whereas

I can babble on about everything. And I didn't want to come off as silly or not intellectual enough to be U of C–worthy. Besides, he made me nervous, and I never wanted to cross the line into flirting.

When Linda and Michael broke up during our second year, he, of course, became the enemy, so we never really hung out again. But whenever I would see him across the Quadrangle, I would wave, still thinking he was the handsomest guy on campus.

Michael

I met Marilu for the first time in October 1970. She remembers the exact date, of course. I remember that I had been invited to a party at my girlfriend's dorm, a party thrown by the resident master. The resident master was a faculty member who lived in a nice apartment in the dormitory and who served as a counselor to the students. Since this was just a couple of weeks into my first year of college, I did not know many people and was only getting used to being in college and living on the South Side of Chicago. I lived in a dorm far away, more in the city and less on the campus. I liked to feel that there was a big difference between my inner-city Boucher Hall and my girlfriend's dorm, Woodward Court. We were more serious over at Boucher and also more worldly, or so we thought. I was riding high having found a girlfriend so soon after getting to campus, and I practically floated through the streets toward the dinner party.

My family on both sides is from Mormon stock; my father and mother were both raised in southern Idaho in or near a town called Preston. Despite the facts that my father was in the Air Force, that

I was born on an Air Force base in southern Illinois, and that I lived in many other places when I was young, I always considered Utah to be my home state, and indeed, Bountiful—where I went to high school—to be my hometown.

My family lived in the DC suburbs of Virginia between the time I was in the fifth and eighth grades. This gave me some sophistication compared to the other kids when we returned to live in Bountiful at the start of ninth grade. My twin brother, Marc, and I caused quite a stir when we showed up at South Davis Junior High School and then later at Centerville Junior High School. Being tall, smart, identical twins with attitude and a veneer of East Coast education set us apart from the other kids in our school.

After we began school, my twin and I realized that it was fine being in Bountiful, but my older brother, Rob, did not find the transition as easy. My little sister, Julie, who was only five at the time, acclimated as any young child would. But I can say that Bountiful was a very distinct place, a closed community of Mormons, and many of the kids were quite sheltered. Moving back to a small town in Utah from the rock-and-roll sixties of the east coast was quite a shock.

The upheavals of the midsixties shaped me as a person. The Vietnam War generated so much angst in society and led to the flowering of a genuine counterculture dominated by the young. The drugs and the music were the obvious manifestations of this culture, but the civil rights movement, female liberation, and sexual awakening were all part of it. Watching all of these forces play out in small-town Mormon Utah was fascinating, as the kids revolted not only against conformity and the Vietnam War but also against their parents, religion, and an insular way of life. And I was a willing participant, having turned fifteen the year of the Summer of

Love. From this contrast, living an interesting life became more important to me than money or career and, along with wanderlust, led me to stray far away from Utah.

When we first moved back to Utah from Virginia in 1966, I was fourteen and still went to church. The Mormon Church encouraged social activities such as dancing, even though they also enforced a strict code of morality on their children. Devout Mormons tend to marry very young, with those still single in their early twenties considered practically over-the-hill. Even now my cousins tend to marry at nineteen or twenty years of age, both the boys and the girls. The only thing that slows down the mating process is the two-year church mission that begins at age eighteen. By the time these young men return from their missions, their girlfriends have waited for two years for their return, and they almost inevitably get married as soon as they get back.

Despite a strict morality and taboo on premarital sex, the young Mormons are very active in sizing up their prospective mates. At age fifteen I quit going to church and fell out with the strictest of the Mormons, but in high school we all were thrown together and had to tolerate one another. So my dating life began with girls who looked at each guy as a prospective husband (even more than usual), and I became very cautious not to get too involved. I was also a shy young man who was awkward around girls, as I had been raised in a male-dominated household with three boys and a girl who was much younger. I did not properly date until I was almost seventeen and only lost my virginity when I dated an older girl from Salt Lake. And so when I got to Chicago, I was not that experienced and still a bit shy and awkward.

All the moving around had given me the ability to adapt to any situation and to make friends easily, which helped in the move to college in Chicago, so different from high school in Utah. It helped me in my long career in shipping and, later, business. And maybe it ultimately helped me to adapt to so many toxic and harsh environments and made me more readily accept stress. I believe that people can get used to just about anything, and I did get used to problems in the family, the pressures of new situations, and the hazards inherent in working manual jobs in trying conditions. Inevitably, this tolerance of stress led me to accept things that I should not have accepted, including the chemical exposures and emotional strains that led to my cancer.

DURING MY FIRST DAYS AT the University of Chicago I was very alone and disoriented. No one in my family had ever graduated from college, and my family was not involved in my choice of a college, nor my preparation for leaving home and matriculating into one of the most demanding academic institutions in the world. When I left home in early September 1970 for Chicago, my parents had been on an extended golf and drinking excursion for half of the summer. Marc had left for college some weeks before, Rob had married and left for New York, and Julie was with my parents. I had arranged transportation through a ride board at the student union of the University of Utah and so set off with a duffel bag and the money I had saved during my summer job for my new life in Chicago.

I got to U of C earlier than the other students and had to talk my way into the dormitory, since I had no other place to stay. As I looked out my dorm window onto the South Side I felt like I was in for a great adventure. I was so excited to be away from home and, finally, at the college of my choice and in control of my own destiny. Once the other students arrived, I soon became friends with my dorm mates and began to haunt the campus where I would spend four years.

A few days into the school year, I went to the college bookstore to get my textbooks. As I was walking through the stacks I spotted a cute blond girl, who spotted me at the same time. After playing a bit of hide-and-seek we finally met at the checkout lane. Her name was Linda, and she was a first-year student from Ohio, starting out in college just like me. She was flirtatious and friendly, and I was ready to make a new friend. We started to date, sweetly and innocently. In fact, she was still a virgin, and I might as well have been, given my lack of experience. She lived in a coed dorm near campus, where I saw how the rest of the first-year students lived. I was in a graduate student dorm with one floor of undergraduates and only a few first-year students. Though we all had single rooms, they were small and used and tattered. It was far from campus and has since been torn down. Linda, on the other hand, lived in a coed dorm with mostly first-year and some second-year students. Her dorm was very different from mine. The kids seemed younger and more superficial. But on the other hand, the guys there were getting laid, and that was what I wanted, too. I began to hang out at Linda's dorm and mooch food off her dining contract at the cafeteria.

One day Linda invited me to a party at the resident master's house. I rang the doorbell and a voluptuous redhead answered the door. She said, "You must be Michael," and called out for Linda. I was surprised that she knew my name, and then she turned and introduced herself as Marilu. She was a big girl. I will always remember that meeting, and not only because I later got to know her so well. The energy and friendliness poured out of her. But by then Linda was next to me and sped me away to meet our hosts.

Linda's and my courtship moved very quickly, perhaps too quickly. Linda wanted to control me, and at first I mistook that for love. Meanwhile, I got to know Marilu better as a friend. I saw the contrast between her honest and loving personality and Linda's possessive behavior. By this time, though, Marilu and Linda were best friends, and I was not strong enough to break up with Linda.

So Linda and I double-dated with Marilu and her high school boyfriend, Steve, who was a nice guy but not the go-getter Marilu was. It seemed natural that Marilu would begin to date other guys on campus and in the city. She talked constantly about the family dance school, something I wish I could have seen back then. The way she talked about her family, I could tell that she loved them very much. She did not depend on college for her social life, which made her very different from the rest of us. But since she was in the dorm with Linda, I would see her often.

In the first bloom of our relationship, Linda and I were close like only two young lovers on their own for the first time can be. After a month or so of dating we decided to go all the way, and so, with some urging from Marilu, Linda went to Billings Hospital and got birth control pills (still quite a new invention at that time). We made love the first time in my dorm room, far away from the prying eyes of her roommate, Kathi, and the gossip ring that was her dorm. It was sweet and loving. I will always be grateful to Linda for our good times together. I tried to be a good boyfriend, but I liked my friends and I liked to party, and this doomed our relationship from an early stage.

I could not help but have a roving eye, as there were many girls on campus and in the city. But I stayed true to Linda through this time and got to know Marilu quite well. Linda and I went to see Marilu perform in the show she was putting on with a friend of hers at the Kingston Mine's Company Store, *Grease*. She talked incessantly about this show, but I am afraid I did not appreciate the importance of it then, or the importance of theater to Marilu. She had friends from all over the city, but she always had time to speak to me, to share things with me, and to make me feel like I was special to her. In our introductory physics class it was clear that we didn't feel like the types to be University of Chicago students. Chicago students were working hard in school, so many on the track to go to graduate school and become professors. Dreaming of theater like Marilu or dreaming of adventure like me was atypical in that time and place. We laughed about the professor after class as I walked her back to her dorm. I was going to see Linda, but wondered why, really. It was easier to talk with Marilu.

What I remember most about Marilu at that time was her energy. Any surprise? She seemed to burst with energy, flying into dance numbers or Broadway show tunes on any pretext whatsoever. So smart, so sassy, so confident! And I remember how much she spoke about her family, her siblings, and her mother. When I heard about the death of her father, who had been gone only ten months when we met, I could not even relate to it. But Marilu was resilient, determined, driven. I think what has made Marilu memorable to so many for so long is her genuine interest in others, her open and direct midwestern nature. Marilu was formidable then, an imposing girl who carried her weight well, with big boobs and bright red hair, set off by blue-green eyes. Anyone could see the beautiful girl working through the loss of her beloved father. And I could feel some energy coming my way from Marilu, as hard as I tried not to feel it.

I came back from summer vacation to my second year of college determined to split up with Linda. I did it right away and with a horrendous show of emotion on her part. I wavered as she screamed and cried and pleaded and cajoled. But I was determined. As was always the case for me, no friendship remained after the breakup, and so I became the enemy for Linda and her friends, including Marilu. Though we saw each other on campus and would wave, Marilu and I respected the girlfriend code. Who knew the code would last thirty years?

By the end of our second year in college I landed with the girl-friend I would date until after college, when the call of the sea made me abandon all my connections. I saw and spoke to Marilu a few times that next year, when she had moved to an apartment with Linda and Kathi. I still remember a crisp fall day on Drexel Avenue when I walked Marilu to her apartment and said goodbye. Little did I know that I would not see her again for eight years.

CHAPTER TWO

1972–1980

Marilu

I left the University of Chicago on Monday, November 27, 1972, when my old buddy Jim Jacobs, the writer of *Grease*, called yet again. This time he said, "Henner! Rehearsals for the National Company of *Grease* start tomorrow, and I've kept your part open for you. If you fly to New York today and audition, I'm sure you'll get it. But you have to come here."

I told him, "Jim, I have two papers due today. I'm on my way to the library right now. And I'm in a play this weekend. There's no way I can fly to New York on such short notice." He said, "Okay. But you're going to be kicking yourself in the ass if you don't do this."

After I hung up the phone and headed to the library, I immediately wondered if I'd just made a huge mistake. Here I was, knowing I wanted nothing more than to be an actress and turning down what could be a huge opportunity. As I approached the library, I saw my car, which I had parked in front of the building. This never happened. It was so hard to find a spot on the street anywhere near my apartment or the library, just two blocks away, that I took it as a sign. I looked at the library, looked at my car, looked at the library, looked at my car, looked at the library, threw my books in the car and drove to O'Hare Airport, where I bought a student standby ticket for $61, hopeful for the career I always wanted.

I auditioned for Marty, got the part, and called my mom telling her I was not at school but in New York and that I would be dropping out of school to pursue my dream. My mother had always wanted me to be an actress, and being a dancing teacher and a creative force of nature herself, she was as thrilled as I knew she would be, even though this was a huge step and a risk I was taking. I stayed with Jim and his girlfriend that night, and the next day I met the rest of the cast, including my future *Taxi* castmate Jeff Conaway, who was playing Danny Zuko; John Travolta, who was playing Doody; and my future *Bloodbrothers* costar Richard Gere, who was rehearsing with our company before he left New York to play Danny in the London company. The entire cast was young and talented, and I couldn't believe what a good luck charm *Grease* had been for me. After that first rehearsal—still wearing the clothes I had worn to the library—the producers gave me fifteen hours to fly back to Chicago, pack up my apartment, find a replacement roommate for Linda and Kathi, drop out of the play I was in, break up with my current boyfriend, slide a note under the bursar's office door saying I was taking a leave of absence, drive up to the Northside to say goodbye to my family, and be back in that same rehearsal room by ten o'clock the next morning. I never looked back.

I was playing Marty, the part I had played in the original Chicago company of *Grease*, but during the Broadway rewrites, Marty had become a sexier, flirtier part, and I was hired with the understanding that I would lose some weight. This was no easy task, being on the road and at the mercy of restaurant food. But I couldn't blame it only on the restaurants. I was the kind of stupid yo-yo dieter who experimented with every type of ridiculous diet that crossed my path, including often buying a pound of my favorite Jarlsberg cheese and eating nothing but that cheese all day. I called it my 1700-Calories-a-Day Diet, and then wondered why I was fat, constipated, and had pimples. I was so stopped up, in fact, that one day after not having gone to the bathroom for seventeen days, I had to go to a clinic where they made me chug four ounces of castor oil. And that still didn't work!

My eating habits were especially terrible during life on the road. There wasn't a Reuben sandwich I met that I didn't love, so of course, I found myself putting on even more weight, even though I'd promised the producers that I'd slim down. Because I always had thin legs, no matter how heavy the rest of me was getting, I could fake it a bit in my costumes. God love the fifties! When I finally made it back to Chicago, for my final stop on the *Grease* tour, a couple I used to babysit for came to see me in the show, and the dad gave it to me straight. On that night, he had the courage to say, "Marilu, you are so talented. And as someone who loves you, I am telling you that if you want to be successful in this business, you must do something about your weight. You deserve to have a big career, and you're not going to have it unless you drop at least twenty-five to thirty pounds."

Believe it or not, this advice hit me like a wrecking ball. I had never before thought about food as contributing to my emotional or physical well-being, much less my career, and rather than being devastated by the truth of what the dad said, I decided to take action. The next day I started writing down everything I ate. I got hold of an old diet brochure and read up on any eating program that might offer some insight. I was determined to pay attention to every piece of food that crossed my lips. I vowed I would try my best to do no more mindless eating or use my emotions as an excuse to act out against my body. I still had a long way to go before I discovered the difference between true health and weight loss, but at least I was on my way.

Within a few months I had my confidence back enough to get cast in my first Broadway show, *Over Here!* with the Andrews Sisters, also starring Treat Williams, Ann Reinking, and, once again, my buddy and sometimes boyfriend John Travolta. I may have been in better shape on Broadway than I was on the road, but it didn't mean my health and weight issues were any less debilitating. Because I loved to eat, I could get talked into any crazy diet and could swing my weight as much as twenty pounds in less than two weeks for an audition or event. It was always three steps forward, two steps back. Five steps forward, six steps back. I knew I hadn't found a healthy way of eating with better food choices that I could live with every day, which is exactly what I (and everyone else) need to live a long and healthy life. I'm always saying that being healthy is not about counting the calories, the carbs, fats, grams, or points of the same old crappy food! If you improve the quality of the food, the quantity takes care of itself. It took me years to figure this out, but at this point, at least I was thirty pounds thinner than when I was in college.

It wasn't just my food that was out of balance, though. In those days, I called myself a POW—a Professional Other Woman—who couldn't seem to find a boyfriend who didn't belong to someone else. It was the seventies and fun to sneak around, and everybody was doing it, but come Sunday morning, there was always that lonely feeling of not really belonging to someone and sharing a life. With my weight and relationship struggles to motivate me, I got into therapy in 1975 and stayed in it for many years with the same wonderful therapist, Dr. Ruth Velikovsky Sharon. Dr. Sharon worked not only with me but also with many family members and friends, including all of my husbands. She and I later wrote the book *I Refuse to Raise a Brat* in 1999 about the dangers of raising children without frustration tolerance and coping skills. Everything Dr. Sharon predicted has come true, as evidenced by today's rampant affluenza culture. It was definitely a book ahead of its time.

Probably more than anything else, being in therapy for so many years taught me how to have all my feelings, but then use judgment when deciding which ones to put into action. I learned how to tolerate an emotion without letting it get the best of me. This came in handy later on when dealing with Michael's health and the public opinions we were bucking up against; there were plenty of times I wanted to argue with someone, but instead kept a cooler head while I waited for time and new research to prove them wrong.

By 1977, I was living in LA, having moved there to costar in the film *Bloodbrothers*—opposite my old *Grease* buddy Richard Gere— and to audition for other movies and sitcoms. At the same time, my mother was suffering through a brutal Chicago winter and battling her rheumatoid arthritis. The stress of my father's death had exacerbated a full-blown inflammatory condition, and it was only during a few short months in 1976 when she was on what she called her arthritis diet that she looked and felt better. It was the first time in my life that I made the connection between what you ate and how you felt, to be filed away until I was ready to take responsibility for the food/health, mind/body connection in my own life.

No matter what the doctors did to her, her body would try to rally. No matter what amount of medicine and needles they stuck into her body, it would try to make sense of it and heal. While watching them poke and prod and X-ray and drill into her head and put her in a halo contraption and rotate her as if she were stuck on a hamster wheel, and hook her up to thirteen machines while draining her lungs into large watercooler-sized jugs that filled up with fluid the color of Hawaiian Punch, I thought, *Can you imagine if you do healthy things for a human body? How much it wants to heal?* I decided then and there that if my mother survived this ordeal, I would learn everything I could about the human body and save her. And if she died, I would do everything to prevent the same fate for my siblings and me and anyone else I loved or could save. And most of all, I would not let my mother's and father's deaths be in vain. I would become a student of health and share what I learned with everyone, starting with my family and friends.

Even without knowing much about health at the time, it was inconceivable to me to think that my mother had been teaching dance in December, had come down with the flu in January, went into the hospital in February, had her leg amputated in April, and died the evening of May 13, 1978, the night before Mother's Day. Three weeks later I was cast in *Taxi* and, just as I had always felt my father was responsible for my getting into the University of Chicago—because it was important to him—I believed that my mom helped me get *Taxi*, because that was important to her.

•   •   •

MY FIRST DAY WORKING ON *Taxi* was July 5, 1978. I had lost weight from the stress of my mother's death, but I was not at all healthy; I was drinking almost two gallons of Tab a day and eating way too much meat, sugar, and dairy. I was swinging my weight pendulum back and forth by starving myself to "look good" on camera for our Friday night tapings, only to pig out all weekend and face Monday morning up ten pounds. I was even smoking, a habit I took up at the request of my mother when I had put on twenty-five pounds in seven weeks my summer before college. But I was determined to change my life—my normal—and embark on a health journey for the sake of my family.

When my father died I ate my feelings; this time I was determined to eat up information instead. I read everything I could get my hands on. I talked to doctors and nutritionists. I went to medical libraries and health food stores and combed the Bodhi Tree, an alternative bookstore, for non-mainstream information. Over time, I even took human anatomy classes at UCLA. Having been dealt the genetic hand of my parents' conditions, I started by studying arthritis and heart disease, only to realize that all disease comes from the same place—an unhealthy and weakened immune system. The more I read, the more I wanted to know about the human body and its amazing ability to heal itself when given the right tools and information. I experimented on myself with everything from macrobiotics to ayurvedic medicine, from Oriental face reading to acupressure point therapy, and I put together a program that I continue to fine-tune even to this day. I finally stopped acting out against my body and never again put on the fifty-four pounds I lost, nor did my health ever suffer like it did when I was getting sick at least four times a year.

In my first health book, *Total Health Makeover*, I outlined the ten steps I took to completely change my health from my typical Midwest diet full of lots of meat, sugar, dairy, and processed food to the plant-based lifestyle I live today. The first step I took was giving up diet soda. I figured I could do anything for three weeks, so I made a deal with myself that I would give up the offending food or beverage for three weeks, and then I would try it again. If, after three weeks, my body could tolerate it, I would go back to it without regret. And if my body found it intolerable, I would permanently give it up.

After three weeks of no Tab, I was salivating to try it again. With the first sip I felt so sick and bloated and it tasted so full of chemicals that I couldn't spit it out fast enough. I never had another diet soda, or any soda, for that matter, again. On August 2, 1979, I had my last piece of meat and didn't even have to try it again three weeks later to know I'd never eat it again. But the one dietary change that had the most impact was, no doubt about it, giving up what had been my favorite food group up until that time—dairy products.

After being told by a nutritionist that I would never truly be healthy until I stopped eating dairy, I started my three-week sabbatical on Wednesday, August 15, 1979. Cheese had been the cornerstone of my diet, and I craved it daily like an addict. When trying it again, I could not believe how bad it instantly made me feel, especially the experience of waking up the next day after trying to digest it all night. I gave up dairy forever when I realized that the only thing dairy is supposed to do is turn a fifty-pound calf into a three-hundred-pound cow in six months. Which then turns into an eight-hundred-pound cow! (So, if those are your aspirations, knock yourself out!) I can honestly say that nothing in my health journey has had as much impact as giving up dairy products. Removing it from your diet changes your body, digestion, breathing, sleeping, senses of smell and taste, and keeps you from snoring or wetting your bed. Seriously.

In a few short months I had learned so much, and there was so much more to learn. The connections between what I ate and how I felt became more and more obvious to me. I started to look at my weight issues with new understanding. Lightbulbs of insights were going off like fireworks, and I was feeling more in control of my mind and body than ever before.

By the end of 1979, I had stopped eating meat, dairy, refined sugar, and most processed foods. I had quit smoking the occasional cigarette and was exercising at least three times a week. I was reading anything I could get my hands on about nutrition and feeling better and better each day that I lived in this new world of awareness. I was definitely getting a grip on my health. But what was next for my love life?

Michael

After graduating from college, I went to New Orleans as part of my calculated plan to never see snow again. The Chicago winters of my college years were tough on me, but I may have overreacted, as I then spent the next fifteen years diving deeper and deeper into the tropics. After my first Mardi Gras at age nineteen, I went to the next six in a row.

I moved to New Orleans with my girlfriend Carol, who had also been to Mardi Gras during college and was happy to move there. After college she had not gotten into the medical school she wanted, and so she put off the process. But when we got to New

Orleans, she went straight to work in a lab and began to dream of medical school again. She soon befriended doctors and other wannabe medical students and went through a process over the next year that sent her back to Chicago, leaving me in New Orleans with our rented house and shelves of college textbooks. I could say that I was hurt, but I had seen this coming. Plus, it left me free to pursue a half-baked scheme to somehow ship out and get to the other side of the world like the ultimate hitchhiker I had become, only this time on a ship.

All my life I have had an obsession with traveling and seeing the world. I remember as a child reading a survey my father had to fill out for his job in the Air Force. The form asked: "Do you want to travel . . . Occasionally, Frequently, or Constantly?" I told my father that he should answer *constantly*, and he told me that no one wanted to travel constantly. But I did, and I did become a constant traveler once I was unleashed into the world. In four years at college I never flew from Utah to Chicago, a trip of fifteen hundred miles. I rode in cars, I rode trains; but when I began to hitchhike, I hit my stride. This was still the hippie era with people wandering around the country, gathering at places like Woodstock and Berkeley. I hitchhiked back and forth from Utah to Chicago, from Chicago to New York, New York to Boston, Boston to Montreal, Montreal back to Chicago, with a stop in Windsor, Ontario, as the border police held a friend and me on suspicion of draft dodging. And this was just one trip in my first year at college. Later I would hitchhike across the country simply to attend a party or to see a friend. The adventure was in getting there, though many a night I stayed up on the side of a lonesome highway for hours waiting for a ride. But in the early seventies a ride always came.

On my first trip to New Orleans, I bought a train ticket to

Kankakee, the first stop south from Chicago, and then hid in the club car all the way down the twenty-hour journey. It was quite a party in that club car, the Mardi Gras special! The porter kindly never asked for my ticket once we left Chicago, and the party continued all night. I landed in New Orleans and fell in love, a love that I have never lost. Seeing the city for the first time through the fog of a hangover is, I suppose, the time-honored way to fall in love with the city that care forgot. For many years, my mailing address was One Shell Square in downtown New Orleans, just up the street from the Superdome.

But where was my center, my balance, my sense of wellness? I had a strong body and my youth, and I used it and pushed it. My love of adventure drove me into hazardous occupations and hard living, but at twenty-two all I could see was the adventure, and I was ready!

When I got to New Orleans, my first goal was to work in the offshore oil fields, but my real priority and dream was to find a profession that would let me travel to the ends of the earth, of both wilderness and civilization. I had a keen appreciation of how short my youth would be, and I wanted to get a lot of living in before I inevitably settled down. And I knew I would settle down, but first I wanted to roam and to look with my own eyes on the wonders of the world.

My first job shipping out of New Orleans was as a galley hand, a kitchen worker. I had no idea what job I was going out for, as I could not understand the man who gave me the job. He said "galley hand" in his lilting Cajun drawl, and for all I knew, he was talking about Sir Galahad. I showed up in Belle Chasse one morning and took a transport van to Venice. There I boarded a crew boat out to the rig, where I was promptly given an apron and told to clean the kitchen.

Not my dream of being a roustabout! But I guess starting as a cabin boy was a time-honored way to go to sea. I spent two weeks on this rig, and you can bet I was ready to get back to shore! The days were long and boring, and I wanted to be one of the guys coming in for meals—not the busboy cleaning up after them. So I made sure my next job was with a drilling company. My first one was known as Rebstock and Reed, working out of Houma, Louisiana.

On the day of my shift I hitched a ride to Houma with a fellow roustabout I had met at the employment office. He was also from up north, so we got along. As we got deeper into Cajun country, we started to hear the sad French songs on the radio and felt more and more like we were going to a foreign country. Finally, we arrived in Houma and got on the crew boat. We went out into the marshes of the Atchafalaya Delta, never leaving sight of land. We came up on the workover rig just as the crews were changing out. We got our bunks, put on our steel-toed boots, and went out to start our twelve-hour shifts.

This rig was populated almost exclusively by French-speaking Cajuns. And they did not appreciate some Yankees coming in and taking jobs from the locals. Most of these guys had grown up on fishing boats; they were skilled in the ways of the sea and also knew their way around oil drilling. They worked us hard, drilling twelve hours straight, loading pipe all night, hauling materials to the drill-ing floor. Working the floor was what made you a roughneck, a moniker you had to earn. Usually, a crew of two or three men assist a driller in working the drilling floor. Just starting out on the rig made me a roustabout, which is a general nautical term for an inex-perienced knucklehead. Those first days on the rig are all about how you work around the drill pipe without getting your head knocked in by a spinning pipe and the headache balls swinging from the

cranes. The job entailed pulling jacks out of the floor that support
the stand of pipe going down deep into the earth. The drill spins,
water and drilling mud gush out of the top of the pipe, and then
another pipe is screwed in and clamped by the jacks, with the drill
bit a mile down turning and churning and driving core samples up
to the surface. Hard to fathom, really, even for the guys on the rigs.
After a few months if you have any moxie for the job, you make
roughneck, which means you can smoke a cigarette and drink a cup
of coffee while swinging a pipe into place and chatting with the
driller about the fishing off Cocodrie. I wanted to make roughneck,
to earn the title, and spending seven long days working my tail off
was a small price to pay. The money was good, if only because we
worked eighty-four hours a week and got lots of overtime pay.

Every seven days we would get changed out and head back to
New Orleans. This usually meant partying, spending our meager
savings on beer in every small town on the way back. I spent my off
time in the French Quarter running around, the days zooming by.
There was lots of interesting sleaze in New Orleans of the midsev-
enties, and it was fun to be a young night owl. At this point I was
changing from the college boy that I had been to the reckless man
that I became. I wanted no part in a relationship after Carol left,
savoring my freedom to explore. Out on the rig, I had noticed that
the big offshore supply boats seemed to be a better fit for me and
they also offered a better chance to see the world. During one of
my weeks off, I found a job with a company with supply boats in the
Gulf of Mexico, the North Sea, and Brazil.

The difference between being at sea and being on an oil rig was
amazing. On our first trip out, we went to the blue waters far out
in the Gulf of Mexico. There we serviced two semi-submersible
deep-water rigs that were exploring the deepest waters ever drilled

at the time. The sky was blue, the water blue-green, and the boat a welcome change from the cruel twelve-hour days of drilling. It was hard work, but the camaraderie of being part of the crew far outweighed the many days at sea and the long stretches of physical toil. The first job on a boat is as an ordinary seaman, or just an ordinary. To first hear the captain say, "Mate, get the ordinaries and go out and secure those lines," made me feel like I was really part of a ship's crew. Working with these sailors, many who had graduated from ordinaries to become ABs, or able-bodied seamen, allowed me to glimpse the way up the ladder to bigger and better jobs. I heard about sailing across the ocean, of sailing in the arctic and the tropics, and I finally began to feel the true romance of the sea.

This was also most likely where I began to accumulate the heavy-metal toxic burden that caused me such grave health issues later. A modern ship or large boat is a metallic environment—maintenance to keep the salt water from rusting away the steel is constant. The chemicals used on board are ubiquitous and noxious, and the safety equipment at that time was nonexistent. Rust needed to be chipped, then the bare metal treated (pickled), then red lead paint applied. The fumes of the chemicals were inescapable; the lead poisoning unavoidable. Mud tanks needed to be cleaned, engine parts soaked in ethylene-based electro cleaner, steel cut with acetylene torches. Though we laughed it off at the time, the poisons were accumulating. Merchant seamen and shipyard workers have high mortality rates, specifically from cancer-related causes.

After my sailing days, I lived in New Orleans and kept in touch with my old shipmates. Many continued to sail while others got jobs ashore in the oil or shipping industries. The water is bad in New Orleans, with petrochemical plants lining the banks of the Mississippi River from Baton Rouge to New Orleans. The rate of cancer is high in this part of the country, and the chemicals are part of the reason, along with the unhealthy diet. As I have followed my friends from this time in my life, so many have come down with one cancer or another, but then, so have others who never went to sea. The modern world is a toxic environment, with everything from nail shops to dry cleaners being cancer-ridden dens. We laughed off the dangers of being at sea, not only the immediate dangers of washing overboard or getting crushed by anchors or ground up by flywheels but also the long-term dangers hidden from us by our youthful folly. This is still true for so many people now in all walks of life, purposefully pursuing those behaviors that will eventually cause them to lose their lives through cancer or heart disease. Often they feel they must perform their jobs at their peril for economic reasons.

AFTER I BEGAN TO SHIP out, I worked the usual seven days on and seven days off. Soon I got assigned to the engine room as a wiper, which is the lowest level on the engine crew. More noxious chemicals awaited me in the engine room—the constant smell of diesel oil, the asbestos-lined exhaust pipes, the toxic waste dump of the bilge water. But in the engine room I found my mentor, an old engineer who needed a young buck to help him stand watch and pull wrenches. He quickly made me an oiler, the next step up the ladder. I took to this assignment with relish, as it ensured a quick ascent up the ranks to the higher pay scale and travel potential of a chief engineer.

I was working for a company named Euro-Pirates International—an eccentric outfit owned by an oil field veteran, Charlie Slater. He had a fleet of twenty-one boats, with some in the

North Sea and the Gulf Coast and a large group in Brazil. Some months after I began in the engine room, the rumors were that some boats were headed north to work in the North Atlantic off New Jersey and Massachusetts. My friendship with a chief engineer named Phil paid off, because when he was sent to Europe to pick up a boat and deliver it to Newport, Rhode Island, he requested I be sent up north to meet the boat and work as his oiler.

Now I had achieved the first part of my dream, to be sent by a company at their expense to a foreign land, but that foreign land happened to be Rhode Island. As we sat in a small shipyard in Newport repairing the MV *Jean Lafitte*, named after the Cajun pirate. I learned so much about ship repair. I had never seen the bottom of a boat before so this dry dock opened my eyes. We had to do a total overhaul to get her ready for duty in the North Atlantic. Because we were laid up in dry dock we had time to see what a foreign land it was.

Newport at that time was a depressing place, though still a beautiful city with a historic colonial downtown and the mansions on the bluffs. It was also an abandoned naval town with high unemployment and lots of angry men looking for work. When they heard about the oil field opening up, they assumed there would be open jobs aplenty for them, as they were fishermen, retired naval personnel, and certified able-bodied seamen. But the Gulf Coast companies preferred their own, so at first they did not hire many locals. We became targets for their wrath, carpetbaggers come to take their due away from them. And we, young and impetuous, fed that fire of resentment by sauntering all over town and chasing the local women.

I had gone from being the outcast Yankee on the Louisiana Gulf Coast to being the carpetbagging non-union scalawag from the South come to take away the work from the Yankees. Luckily, I had learned from my often-uprooted childhood to lose myself in the culture of wherever I happened to be living. My constant shape-shifting kept life interesting.

One night, the chief engineer Phil and I went to the local bar to have some fun. The tension was thick as we ordered drinks with what seemed to be the entire town of young toughs glaring at us from behind their beers. Phil and I were laying it on thick, talking about the boat and the rig and New Orleans and flirting with the bar girls. There was an old jukebox standing against the wall, so I went over and played the Hank Williams song "Why Don't You Love Me Like You Used to Do?" which really infuriated the locals . . . as I had expected that it would. One of the guys went over and canceled my song, and so I went over and played it again. Then the same guy canceled it again, and, of course, I played it again. By the time I got back to my seat at the bar, the place was seething. I turned to the crowd and yelled, "Don't ya'll like country music?" That set them off, and the next thing we knew we had twenty guys fighting to take a swing at us. Now Phil could hold his own—fifteen years on oil boats and he was only thirty. I did my best to keep up with him as we threw guys over the bar and smashed them into tables, but there were twenty of them. Lucky for us the police had gotten wind of the trouble brewing, broke up the melee, and carted us off to jail. And hell, it was the other guys who threw the first punch!

Sitting in the jailhouse, Phil and I had adjoining cells. There was a peephole that connected the cells, so we traded cigarettes and had a good old time laughing about the brawl we had just been in. We were there about an hour when the port captain for Newport showed up with the chief of police and got us out. They apologized and drove us down to the shipyard and warned us not to go back to that bar. Of course we went back, many times, but the locals never bothered us again.

Finally the boat was ready and we began to service a drilling rig northeast of New York City. Even though we were far out to sea, we could see Styrofoam cups and plastic bags floating in our wake. The sky was blue, but even up there, hundreds of miles north of New York, we saw a brown haze on the horizon. Forty years ago the total pollution of our earth was already well advanced. On board the boat we had long days with nothing to do but smoke, drink coffee, and play cards. There was no place to exercise or take a walk; instead we waited for the arrival at location, so we could go outside and work. The food came mostly from cans or was frozen and was often boiled or fried. Unbeknownst to us seamen then, our time at sea was not healthy. The monotony at sea can lead to cabin fever, which makes everyone long for port and the environment that much less healthy.

After a year sailing the North Atlantic, a company boat sank in the Amazon. Soon we were told officially to get ready to go to Salvador, Brazil. I was so excited. This was really the life of a sailor. We all went downtown together to get physicals and some shots, including for malaria and yellow fever. We loaded up with supplies and headed out to sea. We sailed down the middle of the Atlantic, just passing by Bermuda and through three hurricanes, as it was early September in Hurricane Alley. The trip was smooth other than the storms, which battered us and blew us off course, but were nothing more than a nuisance compared to the storms of the North Atlantic. We first spotted Brazil when we saw the city of Recife on the northeast coast—a shimmering mirage of white lying on the blue sea. That same day we came upon fishermen far out to sea on rafts no bigger than picnic tables, standing barefooted and holding their fishing lines, as they surfed along the swells. It was surreal to see how they managed to live at sea with so little equipment. I knew then that I was entering a different world from any that I had known. As we sailed by, the young men looked at us and waved, their smiles huge and welcoming, their hands flat and leathery from days at sea pulling on fishing lines. I wondered how it would be to live like they did, how it felt to be one with the sea. I wanted to sink ever deeper into this new life.

We sailed into the Bay of All Saints on September 15, 1976. I looked at the beautiful city of Salvador, Bahia, with its white buildings from the deck, and wanted so much to climb the hill and see Brazil! The customs inspectors came and cleared us, and we docked at the port in the ancient downtown.

All of the old salts had waxed on about how great Brazil was for a sailor. Beautiful women! Tropical weather. Long idle days in port. Great food and drink. What was not to like? I had been studying Portuguese during our voyage, but it did me little good onshore. The language was beautiful, but incomprehensible. Melodic and singsongy, sure, but I did not get a word of it. I turned on my radio at night and listened to them babble on, and after a while, some of the words stood out from the others. It took me two years, but, eventually, I learned the language better than any of the other American seamen, just enough to get me in trouble.

I met a girl on the beach who was a typical Brazilian beauty, *morena*, as they say in Portuguese, a darkly tanned girl with beautiful brown eyes and black hair. Her name was Mauriceia. I imagined all sorts of things about this girl, and like the good sailor I was, I began to dream of settling down in this sun-kissed spot and giving up the sailing life. Soon she had me tied up, so that none of the other girls dared to talk to me. I loved her then and was happy to feel so wanted, but, in retrospect, I should have taken my time and learned more of the culture before settling down.

We left for a long voyage, then finally after a few months of being at sea we returned to Salvador. My girlfriend had come down to the port each day looking for me, and she was angry that I had been gone so long. But we soon made up. While I was gone I had had time to reflect on this relationship and had come to a decision: I wanted to be with her. So I made more of a commitment than ever and moved her and her young daughter to my next port, Vitória, which was between Salvador and Rio de Janeiro. I was young and in love, and even though there were warning signs aplenty, I ignored them and dedicated myself to making this work. In Vitória, we eventually got pregnant. When she told me, I proposed to her on the spot, as a band played outside in the town square. After only two years in Brazil, I was now married and negotiating the emigration bureaucracy so I could take my new bride to the States. After many delays, I finally got her there when she was eight months pregnant, along with her two-year-old daughter, Carine. We arrived in Utah just in time to have the baby, but we did not have a doctor and ended up in a public hospital, with three different doctors doing duty to deliver my little girl, Cassia.

The idea of bringing my new bride to Utah, eight months pregnant, along with her two-year-old daughter, made sense to me at the time, but looking back on it, it was foolhardy. After all of those years away from home, I soon saw there was nothing left to go back to. Everyone had moved on with their lives, and I felt so out of place. The experience made me feel alienated, though I had, in fact, alienated myself through my constant traveling. I suppressed my feelings and kept my disappointment inside, never expressing it—a lifelong habit of being stoic that led me to suffer in silence. I left Utah with a babe in arms, a toddler, and my disoriented wife for New Orleans and returned to life as a seaman. Again, all of this sailing meant continual exposure to harsh chemicals as well as the rigors of the sea. Eventually I realized it was not fair to my wife to keep sailing and leave her alone with two babies in a strange land. I got a job with another boat company, working out of a port at the mouth of the Amazon River. Belém was a beautiful spot, and for the year we were there, the marriage almost worked. The girls were young and my wife was in her element. She made friends, so it wasn't too bad when I left her and went to sea. The girls were not old enough for school, so there was no responsibility to get them anywhere on time, a problem that proved troublesome as they grew older. The rig was a two-and-a-half-day journey from the port, off of Devil's Island near French Guiana. We crossed the equator on each trip to the rig. After a year, we were sent back to Salvador. Being back where we started did not work for my wife or for me, so we decided to go back to the States again, but this time to the golden land of California to work offshore in the Santa Barbara Channel. I moved the family to Oxnard near Port Hueneme, my new home port. I liked California, but the job was not good, as the rigs were too close to the dock, which meant constant loading and unloading and no cruising time out to the rigs. So I quit the boats for what I thought would be forever and drove my little family all the way back to New Orleans to try to find a job ashore. This was early in 1980.

By this time my girls were getting older and the problems in my marriage more profound. My wife and I didn't share a background or the same ambitions. I hoped that she would learn English and the American way of life, just as I had learned Portuguese and the Brazilian way of life, but this did not happen, and it hurt all of us—my wife, our children, and me.

One day I was in downtown New Orleans walking to an appointment for my new job selling marine coatings and decided to take a shortcut through City Hall. As I walked down the hall toward the exit I heard a voice call from behind me, "Michael!"

1980–1982

Marilu

What was I thinking?

My first husband, Fredric Forrest, and I fell in love at first sight at a screen test for the feature film *Hammett*. I was one of several actresses testing opposite him that day in January 1980, but being the last of six definitely had the advantage of my not knowing there had been a kiss added to the scene. When Freddie kissed me, we couldn't stop, and from this initial spark of chemistry, I got cast to play opposite this Academy Award–nominated actor in a Francis Ford Coppola–produced, Wim Wenders–directed movie. After our auspicious beginning, followed by months of crazy fights, jealous accusations (on his part), and passionate makeups that only confirmed we were wrong for each other, we did what only people in a dysfunctional relationship would do—we got married.

So there we were, less than nine months after the screen test, sitting in a courthouse in New Orleans, waiting to get a marriage license. Neither of us was from the Big Easy, but there just happened to be a special on airfares from Los Angeles to NOLA that month, so we sent sixty-six friends and family members airline tickets and hotel vouchers asking them to "Just show up!"

Tensions between Freddie and me were running high, as they always were when we did anything remotely resembling real life. He and I had very different styles of behavior, especially when it came to making plans. I love and live to organize, and he was more the "let's wing it" type. We were so different, in fact, that my sister had a newspaper printed with the headline, "Desperado Weds Showgirl!" as a bridal shower gift. Two days before the wedding, we were sitting in this tiny room in New Orleans waiting to fill out our marriage license. The room was barely big enough for two chairs against the wall and a small space leading to the clerk's window. Knowing it would be easier for me to figure out what needed to be written since paperwork was much more my thing than it was his—I was always the kind of kid who was banker in Monopoly—I started filling in the marriage license document when Freddie stopped me by saying, "I'm going to fill it in. I'm the man, and this is what men do. My father filled in everything, and if we are going to be married, then this is my job from now on." I sat down and let him have at it. By this time, I'd learned not to fight his irrational pronouncements but rather to wait, knowingly amused that, at some point, I'd have to come to the aid of the clerk who would be trying to help him. Or I'd help him myself, if he'd let me. (It was a lot like that famous scene in *Taxi* when Reverend Jim gets his driver's license.)

Taking my seat, I was, of course, thinking, *This is the craziest thing I've ever done. How could this possibly ever work?* When all of a sudden, I looked to my left out into the courthouse hallway and who should be walking past the doorway looking straight ahead, not glancing into my room or checking out who was in it, but . . .

wait . . . could it be? No. That's crazy. We're not in Chicago. *Is that Michael Brown from the University of Chicago? That had to be. No one else looks like him* . . .

Running out into the hallway, I yelled, "Michael!" loud enough for him to hear me, but not so loud as to draw any more attention than I wanted. After all, my soon-to-be husband was already mad at me for wanting to speed up the paperwork process; I didn't need Freddie to call off the wedding should he take one look at Michael in all his six-foot-three, piercing-blue-eyes splendor.

Michael's and my brief but ultimately meaningful conversation went something like:

ME: What are you doing here?

HIM: I'm just taking a shortcut through the building.

ME: I'm getting a license. I'm getting married!

HIM: I live here now . . .

ME: Want to come to the wedding? It's Sunday!

HIM: Sure. Let me give you my number.

ME: Just tell me. I've got a really good memory.

After giving me his number, we said our goodbyes, and as he walked away, all I could think was, *How come I'm not marrying a guy like that?*

As painful as it is to remember that moment and want to go back in time to reset the course of our history, I'm so glad that the next twenty-two years, five months (minus four days) played out as they did. Michael and I were not ready for each other then. There would have been too many people negatively affected and too many life experiences unrealized had we gotten together when we were both twenty-eight.

Walking back into the marriage license room where Freddie was still trying to do his manly thing, I realized that I'd never make that follow-up call to Michael about the wedding details. I remembered his number, of course, but felt his physical presence alone would be too loaded an issue for my already doomed nuptials, never mind how smart and sweet and interesting I always thought Michael was. Freddie was the most jealous person I'd ever been involved with. And if he'd even taken one look at Michael—never mind that Michael was married with two kids—Freddie would never have stopped torturing me, let alone married me.

Michael

I turned and could not believe I was seeing Marilu Henner standing there with her hands on her hips, staring at me. I walked toward her, and she said, "What are you doing here?" I told her that I had been sailing around the world and had come back to live in New Orleans. "But what are *you* doing here?" I asked.

She told me that she was getting a license to get married in two days. I vaguely knew that she was acting on a TV show, but knew nothing of her personal life, even though she was famous at this point from *Taxi*. She told me that she would invite me to the wedding, and I said, "Great! You want my number?" She said, "Sure, just tell me and I will remember. I have this weird memory." I gave her the number and we said quick goodbyes, as she seemed to be in a hurry to go back into the room to rejoin her fiancé.

I walked out of the building thinking what a small world it was and how strange to meet up with Marilu after all of these years. Being married at this point, and not that happily married, made me think of what I had missed. Marilu looked great, and, in retrospect, I had much more in common with her than I would ever have with my Brazilian wife. I wanted to go to the wedding and see what her life was like. I had picked up some energy from Marilu during our brief encounter and thoughts of all different types raced through my head.

I went home and waited for the phone call from Marilu. I told my wife that we might be going to a wedding reception, but the call never came. I spent a couple of years in New Orleans, working my way up in the business world while sporadically returning to sea. Finally, I hooked up with a marine chemical company that moved us to New York for a year and then to Rio de Janeiro. During those years I often thought about that chance meeting and wondered why Marilu was so happy to see me, but then failed to call. I figured that she had exaggerated her memory and that she should have written my number down.

Marilu

The insanity of my relationship with Freddie only helped solidify my quest for health. Freddie was a man of extremes, and I witnessed firsthand what happens when you live your life that way. He would be completely sober for five days, only to binge drink for three days until he was so sick he couldn't get out of bed for a day, all the while promising, "Never again." Until next time. The following week. As an actor he could change his body for any role he was playing, once putting on twenty-five pounds in less than a month because another character in the movie had the line, "You look like an egg!" A brilliant method actor to the core, he would live, behave, and eat however he thought his current character did.

When we married in 1980, Freddie was aware that I loved to cook tasty, healthy meals that people really seemed to enjoy, but I was not eating meat, poultry, dairy, or sugar. I was plant-based before they even called it that. But that didn't stop him from wanting me to cook a meatloaf because, "Wives should cook their husbands meatloaf," or getting angry when I happily ordered two baked potatoes at a Montana chophouse. His occasional outbursts had less to do with food than with his alcohol-fueled jealousy. But no matter the source, I was determined to become as healthy as I could be. Discovering that centered food equals centered behavior was the key.

When studying macrobiotics, I discovered that not only is your body always looking for balance but also that all foods could be placed on a number line from yin (expansive) to yang (contractive). And all food can be divided into three categories, each having its appropriate place on that number line. The most extreme yin foods are sugar (and other plant derivatives like drugs, alcohol, and coffee), and the most yang foods are salt (and animal foods like meat, poultry, and cheese). In the center of the number line would be the most balanced foods, which are the plant foods like fruits, vegetables, grains, legumes, nuts, and seeds. The more I ate the centered foods—foods placed in the middle of that scale—the more I felt capable of handling anything life threw at me, even in the middle of a crazy marriage. No more cravings for extreme foods. No more swinging my weight pendulum from one extreme to the other. Even my PMS symptoms changed, as I was no longer tempted to give in to the mad cravings I'd get the week before my period. They were gone with better eating. I learned to handle my emotions so well, in fact, that no matter what time of the month, it became obvious to me that Freddie and I could no longer be together. When you get healthy, you cannot tolerate that which is unhealthy.

Freddie and I were married for two painful, tempestuous years, ending with him in AA and me in Al-Anon trying to make sense of it all. Every relationship teaches you what works and what doesn't, and, with Freddie, I learned that marriage shouldn't be about getting to know someone after the fact or trying to change someone for a *better version* of themselves you hope they want, too. And it's *especially* not about taking on the roles you saw your parents play, rather than acting on what *you* do best. That will only doom you from the beginning or allow the universe to send you a glimpse into your future—even if it takes more than twenty-two years for your future to find you again!

CHAPTER THREE

Michael

I moved with my family to Rio de Janeiro in 1983. Being trans-ferred back to Brazil was the fulfillment of a dream, but instead of working on a boat I was starting up a new business as an affiliate of an English chemical company, Perolin. The year my family spent in New York and the first few years we spent in Rio were some of the best times of my marriage. A year after arriving in Rio, my son, Michael, was born. The girls were going to a good American school that catered to ex-patriots, and my business was growing.

Although I was working in the tropics, the days were not full of siestas. Soon after arriving in Rio, my English company merged with a much larger Norwegian company, one that was already well established in Brazil. I was somewhat of an orphan, an American working for an English subsidiary of a Norwegian company. The Norwegians liked to employ their own, and, being from the frozen north, they coveted the manager's job in Rio. The Brazilians took advantage of the Norwegians who were shuttled in and out of Rio every couple of years before they learned the language or the cul-ture. I was a hybrid as I knew the language and was married to a local, but was still an American with a different sensibility toward work and responsibility.

Stress in the company built up over time after the Norwegian boss fired his local manager, who then went to work for the competition. A new Norwegian manager, Lars, was shuttled in, with no notion of the history or of what a corrupt person this fired manager had been. Harassment and threats soon followed, so cruel and unrelenting that poor Lars fled Brazil for the Norwegian consulate in London in a panic, abandoning his job and his company. He even left his car in the short-term parking lot at the airport! I was left to pick up the pieces of this shattered business and deal with the corrupt troublemaker who was still out there, which I did, at a peril to my own life, or so it seemed to the employees I now managed. But the Norwegians never did trust me, and they trusted me less because I was able to handle the strange and savage culture of Brazil. The stress of their resentment and distrust bothered me for the four years that I ran the company.

Meanwhile, my personal life was in a shambles. The vices of the eighties had come to Brazil, and I was sucked in to the partying and drug use. This exacerbated my mood swings and led to horrific fights with my wife. She, for her part, would undermine me with the children, keeping them from school when I traveled. The stress was so great that I herniated a disk while trying to quiet my son on his first day at school, carrying him from building to building, up and down the stairs.

My doctor in Rio, who had been educated at Harvard Medical School, advised me that surgery was indicated for my back, but I refused. He told me that the only alternative was bed rest for six weeks. I chose the bed rest. This time allowed me to reflect on my life and where I was headed. I gave up the partying and dedicated myself anew to my marriage. I tried so hard to be there for my children. But even with the changes in my lifestyle, the marriage was doomed, and, after some time, I saw that the only hope for my family was in bringing them back to the States to try again to live in America.

The bed rest first showed me the power of the body to heal itself. I just could not see the point of being cut open to repair structural damage; it made no sense to me. I was in no hurry to return to a golf course or tennis court. What I wanted was my health to last a lifetime. The bed rest essentially healed my herniated disk, except for a drop foot condition. I had avoided surgery. This first glimpse of natural health stuck with me and influenced me throughout the years until I finally got with Marilu.

After two more years in Rio, I finally arranged to move to Los Angeles on New Year's Day 1990. I chose a neighborhood in the South Bay area, Hermosa Beach, because I thought it would be more comfortable for my Brazilian wife and our Brazilian children. But the problems with my wife and children continued to get worse. The girls were now teenagers, with all of the problems that a toxic home life can give to adolescents. Due to my wife's incessant unhappiness, we moved from house to house, and the girls could never quite get settled. Both Cassia and my son, Michael, were dyslexic, which added to the pressure to nourish them in school. But I was starting a new business and had to travel, and the dysfunction continued, as they missed school whenever I was gone.

Working in a start-up was another source of stress. My brother Marc and I started BrownTrout Publishers in 1986 after he exited a previous publishing venture that had been a partnership with an old friend from junior high school. My brother and I had always loved books. We spent many days of our young lives in used bookstores, collecting old books and reading. The initial company, which published regional books and, later, calendars, was run by an old friend, Ken, with my brother Marc as his partner and sales manager. They created great books, but neither was good at managing a business. This inability to take the financial side of business seriously would eventually doom their first publishing venture, which was doubly a shame because it didn't teach the Browns a lesson: we repeated the mistake with BrownTrout and almost lost our business as a result.

In 1986 I had some excess funds to invest, and when the chance came to start BrownTrout with my brother, I was happy to do it. Somehow I knew that I wanted an exit strategy out of Brazil and thought that this little publishing venture might be the ticket. Marc and his wife, Wendover, ran it by themselves until I came back to the States in 1990.

Once I got into the business full-time, the dynamic was always one of polarization. I was in Los Angeles, my partners in San Francisco. I was naturally the "other," as my partners stuck together because they were husband and wife. The constant travel did not allow me to monitor the business, so I had to rely on my partners. This was also stressful, as I was the one who had actual experience with accounting and budgeting. But the business was growing so fast that many of these problems remained hidden, as growth seemed to cure all ills.

After years of stress, of strain, of trying to make things work, my marriage finally ended with a whimper in 1994. What had been a tempestuous relationship petered out as almost an afterthought. We had moved from a large house in Palos Verdes to a smaller house in Redondo Beach. Because the house was small, I also rented a two-bedroom apartment a block away to use as an office. I moved the family into the house and my office stuff into the apartment, and then took a business trip. When I returned, my clothes were no longer in the house; my wife had moved them to the apartment! At that point, I finally realized how easy it would be to just finish this marriage off once and for all. Before I returned to find my clothes turned out, I'd had no intention of giving up on my married life; I was so dedicated to trying to get my children through school that separation and divorce never really occurred to me. But with this de facto separation, I saw that all I had to do was act on my wife's opening move, and I was gone!

But my children were so lost at that moment. It had not been fair to move them from the only home they had ever really known, Rio de Janeiro, to a place like Los Angeles at the tender ages of fourteen, twelve, and five. The girls were pushed into a middle school environment of competitive kids and straitlaced parents, while my son was only learning English when we made the move. On top of that, the four years after our move to LA were played out in four different houses. By the time we separated, Carine and Cassia were eighteen and sixteen, respectively. Carine was out of school and trying to work and be the adult of the house. Cassia had fled our house for another, and then another, and, finally, left for good with an older man after dropping out of school. My son, Michael, had had a hard time in school, understandable given our tumultuous home life. As I began my life alone, I realized how accustomed I was to being a family man, even in a family that was so dysfunctional. The afternoons and evenings weighed on me. I felt like such a failure. So many years trying to hold together a family that was destroyed from within. The guilt and horror and waste ravaged my mind. I sank into a profound depression. I pulled down the shades and I cried on the couch, and I cried and cried. Nothing could console me. I went days, then weeks, then months living in agony and regret. I had tried so hard to make something work that just would not work. And all of the time I was making it worse for my children, not better!

I have since learned from Marilu that depression is anger turned inward. And yes, I had such a deep anger toward my ex-wife and such regret that it drove me to despair. And this anger and self-loathing not only continued to hurt me for years, it also hurt my son, so young and impressionable. Having to watch his father suffer so and seeing me do nothing to help myself must have profoundly affected him. Because, indeed, I never did do anything to address my depression—I never went to a doctor or a therapist. I just suffered through a nervous breakdown and took my son along for the ride. And although this was nine years before my cancer diagnosis, I believe the seed of my bladder cancer took root then.

I raised my son the next few years, finally ridding myself of the depression and starting a new relationship. My new girlfriend, Gloria, was good with Michael when he was young, and I was glad to have a family again.

Marilu

Perhaps the most important thing I learned from my first marriage to Freddie was that I loved the whole idea of what a marriage *could* be—*if* you marry the right person. I knew I wanted to have children at some point, but never felt the ticking clock until it was almost too late. As I set out on the quest to find my missing piece, I went back to hanging out with my old buddy John Travolta, whom I had dated and lived with on and off during the seventies and eighties. We were great friends with a lot in common, but I always knew deep down that we would never end up together. We were always more like brother and sister than two people who were in love and willing to share a life together. I adored Johnny, and we spent many fun years traveling and sharing lots of compatible career experiences before I knew it was time to think about marriage and having the kids I knew I wanted.

By the mideighties, I was (finally!) in better health than I'd ever been and feeling like I was onto something, not only because of the healthy food choices I continued to make, but also because of the new disciplines I had added to my repertoire. This newfound information included food combining—the art of pairing foods mindfully so that they don't, as I like to say, fight each other in the digestion process. I had learned about food combining in 1980 from reading the book *Ten Talents*, written in 1933, but food combining was made popular again years later with several other books. And in 1981, I also discovered the magic of high colonics, which helped me understand the power of what I like to call *taking out the trash*. No longer needing four ounces of castor oil to get me moving, my food choices were now making it possible for me to have a healthy relationship with my weight—and my colon! Health was on its way, so it was time to think about the family I'd always dreamed of having.

Enter Rob Lieberman.

Rob was a director, producer, and a single father with two wonderful children I got to stepparent, and a man who loved the idea of adding to his family. After dating less than two months, Rob proposed, only to have me answer with a resounding, "No. It's too soon. We haven't even been to Europe yet!" There was no way I was going to make the same mistake I had made the first time by marrying in haste. I was determined to know my partner better. This was not going to be a marriage of passion and drama, but rather one of stability and shared interests. After five years of cohabitation and many trips to Europe under our belt, Rob and I decided to tie the knot and start that family. A few months short of nine years after our very first date, we welcomed our first son, Nick(y), and eighteen months to the day later, our second son, Joey, was born—no complications and super-fast deliveries, despite the fact that I was forty-two and forty-three at their births.

My health journey was never more focused and consistent than when I was pregnant. I never understood why some women choose to fall apart, eat poorly, and gain a huge amount of weight when they're pregnant, rather than thinking of pregnancy and childbirth as something as important as getting in shape for an Olympic feat. After Nicky was born, my first book, an autobiography titled *By All Means Keep On Moving*, came out, and as much as I talked about losing my parents at an early age and being inspired to change my health habits, the book did not tell the whole story of my health journey. I was waiting for the right time to tell that story. Right before Nick turned three and Joey turned eighteen months, I was cast in the Broadway show *Chicago*, playing the female lead Roxie, taking over for Ann Reinking, my former dressing-roommate from *Over Here!* and now a Broadway legend. Annie choreographed *Chicago* in the style of Bob Fosse, the show's original choreographer and director. Annie and Bob were a couple for many years, and when she and I were doing *Over Here!*, I'd water her plants and walk their dog when she went to visit him on location in Miami for the film *Lenny*. There's nothing like reconnecting with an old friend, especially when getting cast in the Tony Award–winning show *Chicago* in 1997 turned out to be a life-changing year in terms of my career, health, and family.

Chicago was such a huge hit that, despite the fact that I had performed on Broadway four other times, nothing gave me Broadway street cred quite like stepping into such a stellar production with an illustrious cast. I got into the best shape of my life and people noticed a difference in me from my days on *Taxi*. My castmates wanted answers as to why this was so, and since I had a book deal to write about my health journey anyway, I began to give seminars between shows to anyone who would listen. I taped these lectures, and after the show, I was so revved up from the Fosse dancing that I would work with a coauthor turning these tapes into my first health book, *Total Health Makeover*. The book's subtitle was *10 Steps to Your B.E.S.T. Body!* The *B.E.S.T.* stood for balance, energy, stamina, and toxin-free, and it focused on the ten most important steps I had taken in my health journey: chemicals, caffeine, sugar, meat, dairy, food combining, fat, exercise and stress, sleep, and gusto! I left *Chicago* in March of '98; the book came out in May and instantly became a *New York Times* bestseller. My whole career took on a different trajectory after that, which continues to this day. Besides getting into great Fosse dancing shape and becoming aware of how other people approached health, as the mom of two young boys who were always with me, I was also learning about children's health and behaviors. By 2001, I had written four more books about health and parenting: *The 30-Day Total Health Makeover*, *I Refuse to Raise a Brat*, *Healthy Life Kitchen*, and *Healthy Kids*.

One night during a performance of *Chicago*, I got a note backstage saying that an old pal of mine from the University of Chicago, Paul Hewitt, was in the audience and wanted to come backstage after the show. Of course, I remembered him, but hadn't seen him or talked to him for twenty-five years. Paul and I had been in a freshman year philosophy class together, and the first day of class, when the professor failed to show, I got up in front of the class and suggested we all introduce ourselves to one another. He teased me about this that whole year, but it bonded us forever. He came backstage and we reminisced about our crazy "where fun goes to die" days at U of C and compared notes about the people we had stayed in touch with over the years. I told him I hadn't stayed close to anyone from back then, except for Linda, my old roommate. She was now a very successful set designer in Chicago, and I would get to see her from time to time when I was in Chicago and at least call her on her birthday, as it's the day before mine. He then said, "It's funny you stayed in touch with Linda. I stayed in touch with Mike. Mike Brown, Linda's old boyfriend. Remember him?"

Paul was sitting on my dressing-room couch. I was sitting at my makeup table, taking off my false eyelashes, when I froze, looking in the mirror. I had not heard Michael's name or thought about him for years. "Wow!" I said. "Mike Brown. How is he?"

Paul explained, "He's done very well. He and his brother have a very successful publishing company. Calendars."

I barely heard what Paul was saying. I was trying to imagine what Michael looked like now, and could only muster, "I always thought he was so smart and very handsome."

Paul then inquired about people he knew in Hollywood that I might also know, and when he mentioned that he'd gone to grade school with Emmy Award–winning writer Richard Kramer, I told him, "Yes! I know him! Richard's fantastic. He and Rob worked together on *thirtysomething* and other things. If you know Richard, then you must know Janet Palmer. They went to grade school together, too!"

Paul beamed. "You know Janet Palmer? I've been in love with her since first grade. She was the prettiest girl in our class."

"Well, she's still pretty. And available now. She's recently divorced. I'll call her and give her your number."

Paul and Janet did get together, and on Tuesday, October 6, 1998, while Paul was in Los Angeles visiting Janet, we planned a big reunion dinner with Janet, Paul, Richard, Rob, and me. It was great to catch up with everyone, and about an hour into the dinner Paul mentioned that he was staying with Mike Brown while he was in town. "Why didn't you ask Michael to come tonight?" I inquired. "It would have been great to see him." Paul said he was going to ask if it was all right, but then thought the dinner was just for the five of us. I was bummed, but somewhat relieved because I knew that I had always had a certain unspoken feeling about Michael.

At this point in our marriage, things were not going well for Rob and me. We were spending more and more time apart, and fighting more and more when we were together. By the time I accepted the National Company of *Annie Get Your Gun* in 2000, I knew we were in trouble, but hoped that whatever time we spent apart would bring us closer together with a new perspective. Rob was generous enough to let me take the boys on the road performing in twenty-two cites over thirty-three weeks—he consistently let me be the primary parent, and for that, I will always be grateful—but in three hundred sixty-five days, the boys and I spent only sixty-eight with Rob. It was not enough time to have a healthy, happy marriage. By the time the tour was over and the boys and I got back to LA, a legal separation was inevitable.

CHAPTER FOUR

Michael

As the nineties came to a close I entered middle age. Like so many American men, I had been polluting myself for years. The toxic waste dump that was my body felt like it was breaking down. To many people I still looked okay, but I did not feel good at all; I was bloated, pale, and my skin was puffy. The hair on my chest was white with some gray and a few strands of sick yellow. I hunched over when I walked. My breath stank. My bloodshot eyes were set off by dark, hanging bags. This was all to be expected, as I did not exercise, I ate too much meat, I drank too much, and I indulged my stress and depressive moods, rather than seeking counseling.

For some reason, I accepted this deterioration of body, mind, and spirit as inevitable. I looked around and saw almost everyone going through the same sad transformation. This attitude permeated everything I did and thought, and it affected those around me. I contributed to the negative atmosphere that was slowly killing me. My children suffered, as I was not leading a balanced life and was a bad example for them. I was still not eating right; I was eating what tasted good, not what was good for me. I ignored the fundamentals of my health, with poor dental care, poor exercise habits, and periods of depression.

But as the new century dawned, I began a voyage of self-discovery that was as profound as it was unexpected. My personal life at this time was still very difficult. I was estranged from my daughter Carine while my daughter Cassia was stuck in a bad marriage. My son was having trouble in high school. If one is only as happy as their unhappiest child, then I was indeed unhappy. The divorce had not really solved anything; my children had been hurt, and I was not able to help them since I was not helping myself. Then one day I noticed a pain in my right big toe. I had felt this type of ache before, on a flight to Europe, in a hotel room in Toronto, during a cab ride in Mexico City. I trudged on with my life and tried to ignore it.

In 2001, the night before my forty-ninth birthday, I was in no mood for a party. But I did have a party at home, a very stressful party with my children and Gloria's children not getting along. When I finally went to bed, I felt like the stress was going to kill me. I could feel the stress working its way through my body—the adrenaline, dread, and acidity mixing together to destroy my night's sleep.

The next day my big toe felt like it was being stabbed with pins. I decided to wear sandals to the office. When I got there, the office was ready to party, but I was still recovering from the trauma of the night before. I walked around the office, dragging my right foot. After much drinking and forced frivolity, I finally headed home. By now my foot was beginning to throb, and I knew that I had come down with my first serious case of gout. I should have seen it coming—my identical twin brother, Marc, had suffered from this malady for years. Gout is a hereditary disease that is caused by excess uric acid in the blood; the condition is helped along by the consumption of rich foods and booze and dehydration. For those suffering from gout, kidney dysfunction causes excess uric acid to sit in the bloodstream. This acid is not absorbed easily, so some of it crystallizes, at which point it is then deposited in the extremities, most commonly the big toe. These crystals build up, and when a trauma occurs, such as the stubbing of the big toe, they inflame. When they inflame to five times their original size and hurt so much that you dream of cutting the toe off, then you know you have gout.

I have found that when you are the most ill is when people around you are the least likely to notice it. Most people notice when you have a head cold or when you are suffering from a hangover. But when it comes to sensing that you are having heart trouble, cancer, or organ malfunction, many just do not see it. When I got home that day, I felt like I was dying. I dragged myself to my bed and flopped down. When I awoke a couple of hours later, my foot was throbbing, the heat was unbearable, and I had a high fever. But the only thing my girlfriend wanted to know was whether or not I wanted something to eat. It took a couple of days for everyone to realize how bad this was going to be. I could not walk. The pain of a bedsheet inadvertently pulled over my toe was enough to make me writhe in pain. The very swelling hurt, as the skin on my toe was stretched so tightly that it seemed like it could not let the pain out, holding it all in for me to experience alone.

I was not able to go to a doctor, as the pain was too great. I got the standard medicine, indomethacin, but it is most effective before an outbreak, not during. Once the attack has happened, the event has to run its course. So I lay there for weeks, nursing my toe, thinking over my life and my options. Once again, as had been the case in Rio with the herniated disk, I found time for myself only when I had a health crisis. The stress in my life was coming from so many directions that I knew not to blame it all on any one thing. I was middle-aged, or so they call it, but it felt like old age. Though I had curbed my drinking—at least from what it had been—I obviously was still drinking too much. My life with Gloria was seriously going downhill, and her inability to put our lives before our grown children meant that a breakup was inevitable. My relationships with my children were strained. And now it seemed as if I had lost my health.

I generally believe that things can be made better, that anything can be improved. Lying in bed, fielding phone calls, soaking my foot in a bucket of ice water, thinking of all the things I must give up forever just to get back to a somewhat healthy, semicomfortable place, all of this was a challenge to my optimistic spirit. No one was encouraging me, and sometimes in life, it is nice to have someone on your side.

But life dragged on, and by the spring of 2001, Gloria and I were still acting like we might work our way through our issues. Then gout came and began to change my perspective on things. As I lay on my bed each day I began to realize that only by making big changes could I actually reverse this aging process that was destroying my life. My doctor knew next to nothing about gout, except how to treat it with drugs, so if I wanted to change, I had to do it myself. I resolved to quit drinking. Abstinence did not stop gout from returning, but it did clear my head. Psychologists often talk about how people enable others to misbehave; Gloria and I had a classic enabling relationship. She would drink and indulge her children, I would drink and smoke dope and indulge my morose side. Not a great way to find balance in one's life.

As I lay on that bed I reflected back on how I got there. My father was an unhappy, sometimes abusive, incurably romantic, tortured man and I was my father's son, through and through. No matter how much my parents fought, how much he hated being stuck as the breadwinner, how much he resented living in small-town Utah, he stayed the course. But his children paid for his distress. He was an abusive tyrant, screaming and belittling everything and everyone in his path. As children we could never answer quickly enough, or correctly enough, to avoid a devastating put-down. We were taught to hide from him, not to breathe in his presence, not to tempt the beast. He traveled a lot for his work, and each of his sons in his own way prayed for him never to return.

We would drive by empty storefronts or phone booths, and I would imagine myself living there, with no one to yell at me. As I got older, I would leave early in the morning and not come back all day long. I would find anything to keep me out of the house. My father always approved if we had a job, so I would find any sort of job to keep myself out of his way. I mowed lawns, shoveled snow, delivered newspapers, worked in a carwash, and worked after school, before school, at night. All the while my resentment built up, and I, seemingly inevitably, became more like my father.

Plus I had chosen the wrong person to be the mother of my children. She was morose and always unhappy. She could be kind in her own way, but between us, we hurt those poor young people who were our children. This I saw so clearly while lying on that bed with gout, and I became ever more determined to change my life. But reminisces can only do good if these memories and observations lead to changes in behavior that actually improve lives. As I lay on that bed recovering from gout, thinking all of these thoughts, I realized that I had to change or lose everything.

When I finally got off that bed after six weeks of convalescence, gout was gone and my head was clear. But I didn't know what to do to change my life. I sort of knew what *not* to do, though. I would not marry Gloria; I would not let that relationship stress me out any longer. I would not allow my health to continue to deteriorate without a fight. But how to start a brand-new life in my late forties? It was harder than I would have ever imagined.

I had been sympathetic to the idea of a plant-based diet for years but had never truly implemented one. This was due partly to my relationship and partly to inertia. I was now free to pursue it, even though I had no specific plan to change my diet. Rich foods are ultimately the culprit that causes gout, so it made sense to cut out red meat, sausage, and other greasy fats. In America, though, when someone becomes a vegetarian, the most common method is to replace meat with cheese. We all know that we should eat mostly vegetables, but it is hard to know how to begin. Cooked vegetables never tasted good to me. Raw vegetables did, but other than salads, I knew nothing about raw food. But I had always loved fruit, eating four or five apples a day as a child. I started going to the supermarket and buying all sorts of pesticide-ridden fruit, which I consumed in copious quantities. I also ate cheese as a meat substitute. In my condition this diet was a terrible choice: I would have been just as well-off eating meat. I was also beginning to drink a lot more water, because gout is also a sign of dehydration. It may not have been the best change, but at least I was moving away from my normal.

As I changed my diet, a real change occurred in my lifestyle. Marilu always says that people do not understand the power of food; I now understand what she means. By changing my diet I signaled to everyone that I was determined to change my life, which sparked shock and resentment from my loved ones. My father could not believe I would not drink with him; my siblings could not believe that I would not eat the meat that I barbecued for them. And I think Gloria understood that finally things were going to change.

I finally broke up with Gloria, but freedom is a hard thing to handle, especially if one is used to living in a family environment. Over time I began to value my freedom and the peace and quiet of being alone. My son was acting out his depression by dropping out of high school, but at the same time, I was reestablishing my relationship with my eldest daughter, Carine, whom I had cut out of my life for more than two years.

Problems in the business arose as we grew bigger and more complex. These issues began just as I was recovering from gout and intensified as I began to urinate blood and, later, was diagnosed with bladder cancer. The changes in my lifestyle pushed me even further away from my partners who, like others, seemed to resent how I was changing.

As I began to reorder my relationships, I started to get an almost perverse pleasure in letting people know where they stood. Maybe I went too far. But I found along the way that nothing is better for the relationships you want to keep than cutting off those that you don't need. I would have never have found Marilu without letting go of Gloria; I would have never gotten the respect from my children if I had not changed my unhealthy lifestyle.

After I had recovered from gout in mid-2001, I went to the bathroom to urinate. As I stood in front of the toilet I felt a strange sensation in my penis. Suddenly a glob of what appeared to be tissue plopped out, and then a stream of red blood mixed with urine. I almost fainted! After filling up the toilet bowl, I flushed it and staggered back to my chair. I felt like my life had changed in that awful moment! Little did I know how truly important that moment was—my body calling out for me to do something about the cancer growing in my bladder, but I couldn't hear it at the time.

I went to my general practitioner, a nice guy whom I had seen for a number of years. I told him about the blood in the urine and asked him what it could be. He said that it could be cancer but doubted that it was. The first time one hears that they might have cancer is a singular moment. I took heart in the fact that he discounted it as a possibility, but I will always remember those words. He then said that the hematuria could have come from a strain, an infection, even from overdosing on vitamin supplements! Though I liked this doctor, his thoughts were very conventional, and they helped sway me into a complacency and inaction that almost killed me.

Onward to a urologist for further testing. Going to a urologist for the first time is like the first time one gets a recruitment letter from the AARP. You realize that you have definitively crossed a line into late middle age. The office is always filled with old people. You can take some solace in being one of the younger patients, but you know that will not last either. Sitting in that room, looking at my compatriots in their wheelchairs, wheezing into the oxygen bottles, stumbling behind their walkers, made me feel very old indeed. I wanted to get up and escape, somehow deny that I was one of them, but the memory of the red blood in the toilet bowl made me stay.

The urologist was as old as most of his patients. He ran through the list of usual questions. I described my symptoms, and he nodded his head. He then ordered me to give a urine sample. When I returned the sample bottle, it looked like it was filled with tomato juice. He studied it and concluded that I might have a kidney stone, a gallstone, a strain, anything and everything except cancer. Thus began months, and then years, of maltreatment and misdiagnoses. I had urine tests, cystoscopies, MRIs, ultrasound exams. Meanwhile,

I would have frequent incidents of blood in my urine that would go on for days. None of the standard care I was getting solved, or even illuminated the truth of, the issue.

While the mystery of blood in the urine continued, life went on. I was now single. I wanted to find a person with whom to share my life. But this time, I meant to do it differently. I realized that all of my life I had allowed myself to be chosen, that I had never actually done the choosing. But now I was middle-aged. My desire to play the field was gone. I had changed my ways, been tamed. But where was the woman who could and would share her life with me?

This lonely void that I had in my life was one I had felt before, but this time I thought I had the strength to go it alone and not have to find another woman right away. This attitude helped me to take my time in my new life and try to enjoy it. I was making lots of money, was independent and single, and only fifty years old. But I felt like an old man, my body still polluted from bad food and bad habits. I had done no detox, no cleansing. I could not deny I was getting older, and that fact helped to keep me from examining myself more closely, to see how my strength and stamina were slipping away, even as I made changes to my diet and lifestyle. The changes were not deep enough, and they were misdirected. By late 2002 I was wearing down, just as I was at the top of my game as a businessman. The changes I had made since the gout attack had been major, but they had not been enough to reverse the decline.

I continued to have incidents of hematuria over the next year. In my folly, though, I had never gotten a second opinion from another doctor. I continued to go to this fool of a urologist who just kept screwing around and getting no results. The explosion in the incidence of bladder cancer the previous twenty years would seem to have made any urologist aware of the symptoms, yet mine remained ignorant! And the cancer is so easy to diagnose with a cystoscopy, which, though unpleasant, is not difficult for the patient. But my doctor just did not see, and I did not ask, and so it went for almost two years.

Yet I must blame myself for the repeated failure to diagnose my disease. How could I have gone nearly two years with this symptom and never sought out a second opinion, or informed myself on the Internet? What was I waiting for? Did I think this bleeding was going to cure itself? It is hard for me to believe that I went so long and did so little, and that carrying around the knowledge that I was hemorrhaging my insides did not drive me crazy. To be responsible for your health, you have to see how you have failed, and I failed miserably in tending to the symptoms that signaled my cancer.

Cancer is called the silent killer, but it could also be called the painless killer. If you can feel the cancer, then you are toast; it is almost as simple as that. If the cancer is so far advanced that you can feel it, then it is so far advanced that you will probably not escape it without life-altering surgery, if you escape it at all. My bladder cancer caused me no pain, just inconvenience. Imagine being at the ball game pissing into the urinal in the men's room, when all of a sudden your neighbors notice a stream of red blood running down the drain! What I thought was tissue that plopped out of my penis that first day was actually coagulated blood, and this happened many more times during those two years. I thought I was pissing out my insides, but somehow I was able to ignore my impending doom.

Four percent of men will get bladder cancer during their lifetime, a bit less for women. And the rate is growing. Everyone knows someone with cancer. It is an epidemic. It is not just a disease of the old or the poor or the unlucky. The causes are known, but the treatment less so. Its symptoms, when they become noticeable to others—like blood in the urine—must be taken seriously. But the system is careless. It misses the obvious. It allows patients to wallow in misery and ignorance. I know because my ignorance almost killed me. I tried in a conventional way—I did go to the doctor, and I did go to a specialist, and I did conscientiously do my tests. But it was not enough. Ultimately, I needed to be responsible for my own health; no one in the system was going be responsible for me. Lucky for me, I got with Marilu and we figured that out just in time.

At this time in 2002 I began to see a therapist, who eventually treated my two daughters and me. I thought he was helping me and asked his advice. This was just before Internet dating became so big, and he told me about an agency in Beverly Hills, Great Expectations. Great Expectations was something very alien to me, as I had never been to a dating service. I went up to Beverly Hills and parked with the valet. I went in to a very nice office space with tall, leggy women selling a dating service to other women and a few men. I met my interviewer, Greta, and I got the feeling that I was being taken in, or flirted with, or both. But I liked it and went along with the gag.

Greta crossed and uncrossed her legs as she very officiously went through the questionnaire I had filled out, asking me to verify each detail. She emphasized to me that I would get many women interested in me, and that it was important that I made myself available to date and put in a real effort. As she told me this, she winked at me. She then told me that the fee was $1,400 for a lifetime membership, and $1,395 for an annual membership. I was too far in at this point and so I said, "Okay, sign me up for life!"

I looked through the picture book and saw many attractive

women. It took me awhile to get around to setting up a date, and before I got a chance to choose anyone, I was inundated with offers. I knew this was because there were ten women for every man using the service, so I was not all that impressed with myself. I then began the series of first dates that soured me on the dating service process. I remember one date where the woman was so angry with men that she challenged me to explain why I was on a date. I got tongue-tied as I tried to explain that I was simply looking for a fun relationship with someone, but it sounded to her like I was just looking for sex. And I was, just not with her! I was not looking only for sex, but it was hard to make that clear during one of these crazy dates.

So the dating service thing was just not working. My sister-in-law Wendover had asked me many years before if there was someone from my past whom I wanted to see again. I thought about it at the time, but could not come up with an answer. Years later, a friend of mine, Paul, had come out to LA. He stayed at my house in Redondo Beach and arranged a date with his girlfriend Janet from the first grade, who happened to be a friend of Marilu's. Hearing about this dinner in Beverly Hills with Marilu and her director husband and Janet and another Hollywood friend, I felt a bit left out again, after missing her first wedding in New Orleans like I had. But I also knew whom I would like to reconnect with, if ever given the chance. Finally, I spoke to Paul about Marilu. He told me that I should contact her, as she had seemed interested in seeing me. When I finally got the number, I again put it away. Months later, I finally called her, on February 22, 2003.

Why had I taken so long to call Marilu? I think I knew that this was a serious step; I just had a feeling. She was the only woman from my past whom I could think of calling, and she lived near me and was not married at that time. I think I realized—deep down—

that this might be it, and I was afraid to take such a decisive step. And I was right, because from the moment of that call nothing for me was ever the same again.

Marilu

After Rob and I filed for divorce on June 7, 2001, I entered what I call the sweepstakes period: dating a lot of different people but there's no clear winner yet, no balloons, confetti, or Ed McMahon knocking at your door. I was not looking to settle down too quickly, because with two kids, it's important to choose someone who is serious. So I went the usual route, hanging out with some old boyfriends in addition to letting friends fix me up on dates. Then my friend Sharon Feldstein treated me to a reading with a psychic, and I asked the psychic about certain people I was already dating. One by one, the psychic said, "No, not that one . . . or that one . . . no, not that one either." And then he said, "It's going to be someone with a name that begins with the letter *M*, could be Mark or Michael or Matthew, and this someone will be everything to you, spiritually, intellectually, physically, and emotionally—the whole package." Needless to say, he got my attention. Everything I've ever wanted in life found in one guy named M . . . something? Is it possible for one man like this to exist in the world? Doesn't Clooney's first name begin with a *G*?

I then asked him about my kids and career issues, and he kept tying these in with the *M*. "He will be within a year of your birth and will be a wonderful stepfather to your children, because he's already raised his own kids and they're older." I finally asked him, "Do I know this guy?" And he told me, "If you do, you've never been with him this way." This psychic's readings were supposed to be good for a year, so I could have happened upon this person anytime in the next 365 days.

That's a pretty good shelf life for a psychic reading, so rather than break up with anyone I was seeing, I would keep the prediction in mind as I met new people. For the next few months, I continued in my sweepstakes period with the letter *M* to guide me like Cinderella's slipper guided Prince Charming. Some *M*s were too young and some were too old, but none were *just* right. Cinderella meets Goldilocks.

Finally on a Saturday afternoon, February 22, 2003, I heard the voicemail that changed my life. It had been ten months since the psychic reading and only two months before its extrasensory expiration date, the ESP EXP date. "Hi, it's Mike Brown, a voice from the past wanting to talk over old times. Give me a call." As soon as I heard his voice I literally slid down the wall I was leaning on, saying out loud, "It's the *M*!"

I called him back immediately and, of course, he didn't answer, so I left a message saying how surprised I was to hear from him after twenty-two years and that I would be around tomorrow to talk. Great, twenty-four hours to be nervous. When we finally talked, I literally twisted my body into a pretzel, so he couldn't detect the nervousness in my voice. I asked him if he were calling me to look for his ex, my old roommate Linda, but he hadn't seen or talked to her for years. He was really calling just for *me*. While we played catch-up, talking about how he got my number from Paul, and how he almost came to the dinner in '98, and the fact that he started a calendar company with his brother, I tried to sense in his voice what his intentions were. Was he being flirty? Did he know I was divorced? Did he really just want to reminisce about the past?

He was chattier than I remembered his being. *Could he really be the M?* I thought. He explained that he also lived in Los Angeles. "Fantastic!" I almost screamed out loud. There was so much to catch up on that we decided to meet for dinner, but then realized we'd have to wait two weeks. I was busy the first week, and he was going out of town the second.

I spent the entire evening googling his company, gathering as much info as I could about him. The next day I called back acting like I couldn't remember (as if!) the name of his company just to hear his voice again. This time he was a little more charming and flirty than our first call. There was definitely chemistry between us, and I was trying to play it cool, which is nearly impossible since my ebullience always gives me away. Throughout our email correspondence over those first few days, it took everything in my power to keep from signing out with little Xs and Os. Actually, I sign *xo* with everyone, even casual acquaintances, but he didn't know that about me yet, and this was too important to blow with an inappropriate emoji. On Wednesday he called to say he wasn't going out of town after all and that we could meet sooner, perhaps Saturday night. The big day arrived: March 1, 2003.

My entire body was levitating. I couldn't believe it. I was finally going to have a date (at least I hoped it was a date) with a man I had known for more than thirty years and had admired from afar, but never dared to even *slightly* twinkle in his direction. I had never really spent any one-on-one time with him, save for a few walks across campus after our physics class.

During our phone conversations that week, I had explained to him a little bit about just how much health was an integral part of my life, and he seemed very interested to learn more. He knew a little about the books I had written but hadn't realized there were seven at that point, most of them about the no-sugar, no-meat, no-dairy way I'd been eating for more than twenty years. He shared a bit about his own health issues and deferred to me as far as picking the restaurant was concerned. I couldn't wait to really talk to him and find out where he was at this time in his life mentally, emotionally, and physically. What did he look like after all these years? Would I have recognized him if we had just bumped into each other again? I couldn't wait to hear about his health journey and read his face to figure out how I could help him with everything I'd learned over the years. (This wasn't just a date; it was a diagnosis!)

I carefully chose my outfit that night for a few reasons, not the least of which was that I was twenty pounds lighter than the last time he saw me in New Orleans and forty-five pounds lighter than he might have remembered me from college. I also didn't want to dress too provocatively. Sexy and comfortable, yes, but with the easy access of a skirt or dress, no. I decided on the textures and ease of pants and a top, just in case at some point in the evening we would be rolling around all over each other.

Standing in my kitchen waiting for Michael to show up, I flashed on how crazy it was that we were reconnecting, of course, but even crazier was how positive I was feeling that . . . this was it! He was the *one*—the person I had been waiting for my whole life. The man I had always thought was out there during the loneliest times in both of my marriages. The love of my life whom I had cried about not having when I stood in the middle of a Hallmark store trying to pick out a Valentine's Day card for one of my former husbands.

Michael was forty minutes late that very first date, but I chalked it up to the distances between our neighborhoods. (Little did I know that he was on what I've learned to affectionately call *Brown time*.) As soon as he got out of the car, and I could see him through the window, I had two thoughts as he walked toward my house: *Oh my God I forgot how blue his eyes were,* and *Oh my God I immediately have to get him to my friend MaryAnn for a haircut!* The makeover was on, and we hadn't even made eye contact yet.

He was dressed in pleated beige pants and a blousy, silk, cream-on-beige striped shirt—nice textures, but horrible colors for his skin tone—and unlike anything he's ever worn since, even though the outfit still hangs in our shared closet for sentimental reasons.

When I opened the door, we smiled and gave each other a fast, warm hug where I could actually feel my heart pounding through my blouse. Nicky was eight and three-quarters and Joey was seven and one-quarter at the time, and both came to the door with me to meet Mommy's college friend. As we gave him a tour of the house, going from room to room, I could feel a certain energy between us. We kept looking at each other as if to say, *Wow, is it really you?* I definitely knew he was interested when, walking up the stairs, I turned long enough to catch him looking at my ass. He smiled because he knew he had been busted.

After saying good night to the boys and their babysitter, I got into his car and leaned over to let him into his side, and it felt like the most natural thing in the world to be with him.

The restaurant I chose was Les Deux Cafes, a Hollywood mainstay that, unfortunately, no longer exists, but was quite beautiful and intimate. We would be left alone and, most important, be able to hear each other, which is not always possible in a Hollywood hotspot.

As soon as we sat down, I immediately noticed that I was in the bad lighting seat. There is such a seat, believe me. It's the one where the light source is directly above you, giving you horrible shadows on your face, or it's behind you giving no light to your face, but lovingly bathing your dinner companion with flattering light. I wanted Michael's seat, so I made some lame excuse about wanting to sit and face the fewest number of people, which never really matters to me. But I had to come up with whatever reason for switching I could think of, because there was no way I was going to sit in the bad lighting seat after waiting thirty-three years to sit across from Michael Brown. (Who's in charge of the makeovers around here, anyway?)

After swapping seats I figured, *What the hell? I am going to ask him any question that's been on my mind.* There's nothing like that small window of opportunity before you admit your feelings or even know whether or not the two of you are going to be something, in which you can ask any question you want.

So I asked everything from *Why did your marriage break up?* to *What is your family like?* to *What are you looking for now in your life?* I felt no question was off-limits, because, after all, we were old friends catching up, even though I knew my legs were trembling under the table, and no matter how much wine I was trying not to consume, I wanted to seem casual as opposed to planning our future. We spoke of our children and their personalities and stories. I found out that, even though Michael and I are the same age, his granddaughter, Victoria, was the same age as my Joey. He had married young and had two of his kids before I had even married for the first time. His daughters were twenty-six and twenty-four, and his son was eighteen. As I listened to his stories of family life, I couldn't help but flash back on what the psychic had predicted down to his age being within a year of mine, his children being older than mine, and my knowing him before but never having been with him that way.

Here was the *M*, indeed.

But I still wasn't sure whether or not he thought this was a date. At least until he told me that his girls were excited for him and had picked out his clothes. He was smiling as he said this, and I could see in his smile that he, too, felt this was the start of something special. He showed me pictures and talked about his life after the University of Chicago. How he'd traveled the world as a merchant seaman and landed in Brazil, where he'd married and lived for ten years before coming to Los Angeles. He spoke of the hardships he'd been through raising his kids and the depression of divorce. How his last relationship didn't work out and why. He looked me in the eye and said, "I come with a lot of baggage." And all I could think of was, *I don't care. I'm healthy. I'm strong. I've been through a lot myself. And I've had lots of therapy. Bring on the baggage. You're the M!*

I shared with him my stories of two kids, two divorces, and the ups and downs of show business. We spoke like two people who had known each other a long time but had never really come together as friends. And more than friends: our body language vibrated with the promise of longtime lovers.

Trying to be casual, I excused myself to hit the ladies' room and call MaryAnn, not only to warn her of the mullet she'd have to take care of ASAP but also to tell her, "This is *definitely* a date!"

We sat and talked for four and a half hours and then headed to my house; I was already trying to figure out where we could fool around without the boys waking up and catching us. Since my divorce, I hadn't brought a date home while the boys were in the house, but I had the feeling this would be the first of many nights with Michael, so I wanted us to be careful and respectful of my being a mom. All this was going through my head, and we hadn't even kissed yet! In typical girl fashion, I was already imagining him in my home while he, as he later admitted, was imagining me in his bed.

After relieving the sitter—someone who knew me well and winked as she closed the door—Michael and I opened another bottle of wine and sat in my kitchen to continue our conversation. The view from my home is spectacular, looking down, in fact, at the restaurant that's considered to have the best view in LA. I couldn't wait to show it to Michael, not because he was a geography major but because it seemed the perfect location for our first kiss. Believe it or not, it took us three times looking at that damn view before he got the message, something I torture him about to this day. But once we started kissing, we couldn't stop. We made out like two teenagers, fully clothed, but full of passion, and every once in a while, we would pull apart and look at each other as if to say, *Is it really you?*

After all these years, it was really him. And it was really me. And we both just knew.

As our four-and-a-half-hour dinner was turning into an additional four-and-a-half-hour date, the phone rang with the news that my niece Lizzy was going into labor with her son Jackson. He'll always be as old as Michael's and my relationship. And over the years, Michael and I have looked at Jackson and said things like, "Oh look! Now we're walking!" Or, "Wow! We're starting first grade already!" (Now it's, "He sounds like a man!") But after making out in my kitchen for a few hours and setting a plan for Monday night, Michael left at four a.m. Two hours of happy sleep later, I left for the hospital to be with my sister JoAnn and niece Lizzy at Jackson's birth. When I walked into the delivery room, I announced to JoAnn and Lizzy and anyone else who would listen that I was with the love of my life last night and that *this is it*! I was going to spend the rest of my life with this guy and I knew he felt the same way.

They all looked at me like I was nuts (because it does sound a little crazy, even now), but I knew then like I know now: Michael is the love of my life, and everything else in our lives led up to our being together. This, of course, was all being discussed in between Lizzy's pushing out a beautiful baby boy! We were all flying high that day because, let's face it, there's nothing more magical than the birth of a child. Couple that with a nine-hour reunion date topped off with a sexy make-out session and I was off the charts.

I couldn't wait to talk to Michael again, and I trusted the relationship enough not to stand on ceremony as to who should call whom first, but I didn't have to worry; Michael called at eleven a.m. with a "Wow!" as in, *What was that? And when can we have more of it?* We were both a little giddy with excitement and looking forward to our second date the following evening. The promise of another great night with an even happier ending was in the works—that is, if I could pull it off without the boys catching us. It's one thing to make out fully clothed in the kitchen with enough time to pull yourself together should you hear the patter of little feet on the stairs. It's another to be caught in the middle of what I had in mind for our first time together.

I had to figure all that out before our next date, but for now, I just wanted to bask in the sound of Michael's voice and his sexy way of saying, "Good morning" and "How's it going at the hospital?" and "How great was last night?" I knew we weren't going to see each other that evening, because I was busy with family and he had a good-bye "date"—his last with anyone but me for the rest of his life. That's how confident we were from the beginning. We both trusted that this was it and there were no games, no holding back, no being cool. It just *was*. We were home.

Michael

What made me call that day? Marilu has asked me that so many times. I always reply, "The time was right," which it was, but I had no way to know that before I dialed. I had been single for a while and things were not going the way that I wanted. I needed something more. And somehow my instincts were not so dull. Lucky for me, I figured out my next move in time, because Marilu is a girl who loves options, and I had only a short window of opportunity before she might be taken.

I was surprised when I came back from an errand and found a message already on my machine. It was Marilu with a very sweet and warm message. It was already evening, so I decided to call her the next day. I thought I was being polite, but I was, in fact, being dense.

We soon talked and set up our first meeting. The day of the dinner my daughters were both at my house, which was unusual. Cassia, twenty-four, was living with her daughter very close to me, while Carine, at twenty-six, was visiting. I told them about my date and they got excited and wanted to help pick out my clothes. This was sweet of them, but they picked out clothes that I would not ordinarily wear: hopsack pants and a silk shirt. Thus garbed I headed up to the Hollywood Hills to see Marilu.

Traffic was heavy that evening. This was still in the day of Thomas Guides and Rand McNally. I took my map out and got off at the Hollywood Bowl, then began the long climb up the hill to her house. As I drove up the winding street I thought that this might not be the last time I took this route. Marilu had been very friendly on the phone and once we had gotten over the foolishness about whether or not I was looking for my ex-girlfriend Linda, things seemed to flow very well.

I arrived and drove down her driveway, as she had instructed. I got out and realized that I was almost an hour late, a big sin with Marilu. I quickly apologized as she led me to the house. As I walked in, there was Bel, Marilu's helper, in the kitchen. Nicky and Joey were introduced and I was shown around the house by Nicky. I had a great view of my hostess as I followed her up the stairs; I did not care if she knew. Soon we were in my car and on our way back down the hill to go to the restaurant.

Marilu looked great; I was amazed at how young and healthy she looked. She has long dancer legs and a great body, smooth skin, and beautiful eyes. It was hard to believe I never chased after her before, but that was so long ago. I had to remind myself to stay in the present.

As we drove to dinner, Marilu asked me if I had ever thought back in the day that I could afford a car like the one I was driving. I laughed and said they did not have cars like this one back in 1970. I felt a genuine warmth and curiosity coming from her; little did I know that she is famous for giving warm attention to everyone. Regardless, I felt so comfortable with Marilu even before we got to the restaurant.

The place was very quiet, as I remember it, but it could have been a madhouse for all I knew. I was locked in a conversation, a search with Marilu through our joint pasts and tangled presents. She was recently divorced with two fairly young children. I was a young grandfather and a somewhat empty nester, though both daughters lived nearby and my son was still a teenager. I had such a long story of places I had been and things that I had done, while Marilu's journey was both fascinating and impressive in so many ways. Through a bottle of wine and then another, we talked. Marilu would go to the ladies' room every half hour, while I would get a chance to collect myself and think about how this date was going. Finally I paid the tab and we left the restaurant.

I drove us home, and I was lucky that it was only a few blocks. Marilu had asked me to come in, but then made me be very quiet as we closed the doors to the kitchen and I opened one more bottle of wine. We continued to pour out our life stories along with the wine, though I think she was getting more out of me than I was out of her. I had told her at the restaurant that I came with a lot of baggage, and, indeed, I did and still do. I had learned so much from all I had been through, but that did not mean that I didn't have more things to learn. That I was, at heart, a family man, despite my wild past, and that I had spent more than twenty years raising children.

Why I had told her all that so quickly I couldn't tell you, perhaps to impress her with my honesty. I had been away from Marilu too long not to take the chance now to get to know her. We continued to talk and moved to the couch. She took me to the balcony to look at the view, and, finally, on the third try I got up the courage to kiss her. Why did it take me so long? Because I knew that this kiss meant something; it was a kiss I could not take back. I was falling head over heels in love with someone I had vaguely yearned for all of my life. And I knew it. I had known since our first phone call a week before.

This was the real thing, a prolonged, deep seduction, with my leading her down a road I had longed to go for many years. I held her, kissed her, then pulled back to look at her. The girlfriend code had been broken, the taboo lifted. After the near miss in New Orleans and a wait longer than the Trojan War, we were finally together.

By four a.m. it was time to end the night, but not before making a plan for Monday evening. Marilu had to get a few hours sleep before going to see her niece, who was giving birth to her son. I rose from the couch and kissed Marilu goodbye and then walked to my car. I had just made out with my ex-girlfriend's best friend, with a girl I had known for more than thirty years, and it was good. It was very good! I was awash in emotion as I drove the hour to my house at the beach. I tried to go to sleep but could not stop dreaming of Marilu. I took my dog, Pablo, for a walk in the neighborhood, climbing the hill and the steps of the library, where I sat down with my dog and allowed my mind to wander. My body ached for my new lover; my eyes saw her every time I closed them. I was in that moment of physical ecstasy where desire takes over. Before I knew what had happened I was in love!

The next day, Monday, Marilu and I were to meet again. I wanted to make a good impression and to show her that I knew that this was a date. I went to a florist near my house and ordered some flowers. I told the girls at the florist that this was important, because "Tonight's the night!" which I thought and hoped it was. I imagined that I was now going to see the love of my life; I was not going out, I was coming home. I made my way up to Hollywood and again drove that winding street up to Marilu's house. Marilu is very much a girly girl. She wants to be treated like a lady, she wants to enjoy the interaction between male and female, she wants to play the game. Nicky and Joey almost fell backward when they saw me with the bouquet of flowers, but when Marilu grabbed them and put them in a vase I was glad that I had brought them. Thus began my whirlwind courtship of Marilu.

CHAPTER FIVE

March 3–9, 2003

Marilu

Now *that's more like it,* I thought when Michael showed up for our second date. And it wasn't because he was carrying flowers, which literally made both boys jump back in surprise. *Mommy's college friend brought flowers. What does* that *mean?* I could practically see their thoughts spinning. Michael was wearing black jeans and a black T-shirt and a black leather jacket and looked a lot more comfortable in his skin than when he'd been wearing the clothes his girls had picked out. He had the same goofy mullet, but the hair appointment was already booked for the next day under the guise of a birthday gift, as this was the night before his birthday, March 4. (As Michael always says, "It's the only imperative command in the calendar!")

My wardrobe was definitely different that night, too. Instead of wearing something that was perfect for rolling around, it was time to pull out all the stops with a sexy black dress and heels, and the perfect underwear to eventually look good on the floor. After all, this was the night! No turning back now. And I couldn't wait to be with him in my home. His house was too far away to go there, and the babysitter had to go home, anyway. I just wasn't sure *where* in my house we could be together without getting caught by the boys.

And then it hit me.

My downstairs office can be accessed only two ways: through a double-locked door, or from my bedroom above, which can also be locked. Perfect! Even if the kids yelled out for me or knocked, there would be plenty of time to pull it together.

But there was to be a dinner before the deed at another Hollywood haunt, Pinot Hollywood, where the ambience was sexy and the lighting was perfect. We sat super close to each other, practically on one seat, and laughed about how much had changed in our restaurant demeanor in just two days. No longer the shy, questioning looks into each other's eyes; these were the stares of two equals—people who had been through a lot to get to this place of peace and, soon, passion. Michael paid the check and we headed for the house, both excited and a little nervous about what was next.

I led Michael to the downstairs office with its big comfy couch and went to check on the boys, who were being unconsciously cooperative by being fast asleep. Making sure they were both well blanketed and happy in REM, I tiptoed off to the office, carefully locking both doors between the boys' room and where I had left Michael waiting for me.

He looked so comfortable being in my house. His eyes were twinkling with the look of love and a big smile on his face. It was hard to believe that we'd known each other for more than thirty years. It was all so natural and easy, and I couldn't believe how organically our bodies connected—twice—known from then on as the "first time double dip!"

It was too soon for Michael to sleep over, so as hard as it was to say goodbye that night, I knew I'd see him the next day—his birthday! My present to him—besides what he had gotten from me the night before—was (finally!) a haircut from my BFF, MaryAnn Hennings (although it was more like *my* gift to *me*). I've known MaryAnn since 1983, and I never turn anyone on to her extraordinary hair-styling skills unless I know I want them in my life forever. (In LA, hairstylists and psychics are like family.) I wanted Michael in my life forever, and I couldn't take the mullet anymore, but I wanted more than a sexy night and a better haircut, and my birthday card to him reflected that.

On the cover of the card, there were all these healthy foods with the caption:

EAT A HEALTHY DIET

EXERCISE REGULARLY

GET PLENTY OF REST

And when you opened the card, it actually said:

I'VE GOT BIG PLANS FOR YOUR BODY

And I did. I planned on turning him on to the healthy food that made it possible for me to lose fifty-four pounds, lower my cholesterol more than one hundred points, and have two healthy children at forty-two and forty-three years old. I planned on cooking for him and teaching him everything I'd learned over time about living a healthy lifestyle. And I planned on loving him throughout many years filled with lots of laughs and crazy wild sex. Big plans, but all doable because of good health and a scrappy attitude.

And inside the card, I wrote:

THERE'S SO MUCH TO SAY. I CAN'T WAIT TO SAY IT.

I already knew I loved him. Not just because he was handsome and smart and kind and a great family man and listener and lover and we shared a history. I also loved him because, as my brother Lorin always says, "Women choose men for their makeover potential." And here was a guy who had a lot of MP!

MaryAnn worked her magic on Michael's hair and he was more gorgeous than ever. My housekeeper, Elena, took the boys on an after-school field trip so that Michael and I could have a birthday afternoon tryst in the glorious magic hour lighting, on a real bed this time, and it was even more special and personal than our first time. It was especially intense because we knew we wouldn't see each other for a few days. Michael was leaving the next day for a family funeral in Salt Lake City, and I was leaving for San Francisco to shoot an infomercial based on the principles first explained in my bestselling book *Total Health Makeover*.

I was then, and continue to be, trying to help people live healthier lives. I saw what killed my parents, and I love to share the information that changed my life. Each year I learn more about the human body and how much it wants to heal itself without having to resort to medicine and procedures that interfere with the body's own self-preservation mechanisms. I really do believe we are going to look back on this as the dark ages of medicine. At some point, we are going to say to ourselves, *Wait, wait. You mean we used to burn,*

cut, cauterize, and chemically poison sick people? Suppressing their bodies'
immune system and expect it to heal? What were we thinking?

And that's when you are trying to save a life!

But even when you're just trying to lose weight and feel better,
there's so much misinformation out there, so much noise to get
through. It took me eight years of experimentation, but once I
found a way to eat and take care of myself, and I was able to live
with a protocol I put together over a period of time *every single day*,
no matter where I was or what I was doing. There was no turning
back. I never gained back the fifty-four pounds I had lost, and my
blood work panel has been in the healthy range—which is even nar-
rower than the "normal range"—for more than thirty years. Once
I experimented on myself, I was anxious to share it with others
and wrote my first *New York Times* bestseller, *Total Health Make-*
over, followed by *The 30-Day Total Health Makeover*. The weekend
after Michael and I started seeing each other, I was in San Francisco
shooting the infomercial version for *The 30-Day Total Health Make-*
over called "Body Victory." This was an infomercial that featured
several people whose lives had been transformed by the information in the blue book, as it's called. We were all meeting up in San
Francisco for a few days to shoot their testimonials, as some of the
women had lost fifty-plus pounds by seeing their lives—most for
the very first time—through the prism of health.

There's nothing like the spark of a new love to give you that
sparkle, which is how I felt being in San Francisco, meeting all
these fabulous women and hanging out with my two best friends,
MaryAnn (who was doing everyone's hair for the shoot, of course)
and Sharon Feldstein (who was doing everyone's wardrobe). Both
MaryAnn and Sharon have known me since the eighties and have
seen many boyfriends and husbands come and go. They couldn't

believe how serious-minded I was talking about Michael's and my future the whole weekend, but they couldn't be that surprised considering MaryAnn had already met him, and it was Sharon's psychic that had predicted the *M*!

The weekend was action-packed and full of wonderful moments, but I couldn't wait to get back to Los Angeles and Michael. We had arranged it so that he would pick me up at LAX, meeting Sharon and seeing MaryAnn again, and then we would go to his house in Palos Verdes to spend our first overnight together. The boys were already spending the weekend with my ex Rob, so it was not only the perfect opportunity for us to spend unrushed couple-time together, it would also give me the chance to see where and how he lived, thereby determining how difficult it would be for me to pull him away from whatever I discovered. First the makeover; then the transplant. As a mom of two school-age boys living in the Hollywood Hills, I knew we weren't going to move into his home; he'd eventually have to move in with us.

I know. Big plans for a couple who had their first date only the week before. But that's how sure I was that this was the real deal and for keeps. I was so sure, in fact, that after Michael picked me up at LAX (looking handsomer than ever and charming both MaryAnn and Sharon) and drove to the top of Palos Verdes to show me the majestic view of LA, I told him. I told him point blank that I loved him and I knew we were going to spend the rest of our lives together.

In typical guy fashion—and to this day I torture him about it, much like our first kiss—he didn't say it back. (What is it about Michael's reluctance to express himself when there's a view involved?) But I didn't care. I often feel ten steps ahead of most people's normal behavior, because, having the memory I have, I feel I can see patterns and forecasts that others often miss. Besides, I innately trusted how he felt about me and chalked up his reticence to his not being the extrovert I am, because—let's face it— who is?

The whole night I was analyzing and comparing our homes to be sure he could be happy once he moved in with us. I sound so devious as I write this, but I was a woman with a mission. Michael's house was situated on a corner that had a view to rival mine, so I knew he liked views. (Check.) When we pulled up to the house, a plumber was just leaving and told us that he fixed the toilet, but couldn't fix the shower. (Not a perfect house—check.) We walked in and the house smelled unmistakably like "big dog," and so I met Pablo, Michael's German shepherd who weighed almost as much as I did. (The boys will love having a dog—check.) The house wasn't messy as much as it was "guy" and needed a woman's touch. The bones of it were good, but it really needed a page-one rewrite, which made me happy, because I would have hated to take him away from a newly put-together, well-designed home. Each room screamed *bachelor*, from the large pool table in the living room with a picture of the Rat Pack over the bar, to the mismatched faded towels hanging over the kitty litter box in the bathroom. But nothing spoke to my makeover-loving heart like Michael's bedroom. Nothing matched or fit. The curtains were not on their rods, so they couldn't hang together or close. The bedspread was out of a roadside motel, and the polyester sheets felt like you were sleeping on a shower curtain. I sized all of this up within two minutes of walking into the room, and I knew I could take him away from all of this without any hesitation. (Check.)

Michael had gone to Costco that day to get dog food, socks,

and underwear, and he also picked up Al Green's *Greatest Hits* CD, which he started up as I sat on his barely made bed. To the strains of "I'm So Tired of Being Alone" we danced for the very first time around his bedroom, holding each other tight, the irony of the song title not lost on either of us. By the time we got to the sixth cut, "Let's Stay Together," I was already wondering if this should be our wedding song. (Girls are crazy, aren't we?) We didn't make it through the whole album before our clothes were off and we were sliding (literally) all over the polyester sheets. Despite the lumpy bed and cheap hotel pillows, we fell asleep madly in love with the promise of a sexy second round in the morning.

But I couldn't help notice how Michael's chest hair had a strange yellow-colored patch, which is called a *liver dump* by people who recognize that when your liver is working hard to metabolize the toxins it's been trying to filter, it presents itself through the hair with a yellow color. Michael's liver was definitely compromised, that I could see. And I could also tell how difficult it was for him to sleep and how labored his breathing was. *That's okay. I'll get him off dairy, no problem*, I thought as I tried to fall back to sleep. But this was more than the too-much-dairy snoring I've heard from people over the years; this was deeper and more alarming. It had a more respiratory resonance than just a stuffy-nose sound. But like Scarlett O'Hara, I thought, *Tomorrow is another day. One makeover at a time. Get him off dairy first, and then let's hear what he sounds like.*

I finally fell asleep in his arms, knowing I was in love and that a great life was ahead for us . . . as well as a very sexy morning, indeed.

March 9–23, 2003

The two weeks following our first sleepover could have been a movie montage starting with tuxedo shopping in Beverly Hills (unusual for a guy who buys his underwear at Costco) for our first Hollywood outing—a huge ABC fiftieth anniversary event. I was proud to show off my handsome date, especially after MaryAnn came to the house once again to do her magic. It was not only our first limo ride and red carpet together, it was also the first time Michael was exposed to hundreds of stars all at once, and I wondered how he'd handle it.

I learned quickly that Michael, who had lived in Brazil for so many years, recognized very few stars, unless, of course, they were on *Bonanza* or *Gunsmoke*. (To this day, I call him Rip Van Winkle when it comes to seventies and eighties pop culture.) But that night he recognized John Ritter and Wayne Brady, two great guys whom I'd known for a while, and they both couldn't have been more gracious. I had been on Wayne's talk show several times and always had a great time. And John and I had known each other since 1977 when, along with Robin Williams, we were in an improv class together—can you imagine?—right before Robin got *Mork and Mindy* and I got *Taxi*. John was already a famously huge star from *Three's Company* and was known for being one of the nicest guys in Hollywood. I got to witness John's greatness firsthand in '91 when he and I spent several months filming *Noises Off* alongside Michael Caine, Carol Burnett, and Christopher Reeve. The shoot was difficult, but fun, and to this day, we all feel as though we had been through a war together. John greeted me in his usual hilarious way, and made some comment about Michael's looking like a movie star, which put him at ease and made him feel welcome among Hollywood luminaries. (Many people commented on Michael's movie star or mogul looks that evening, as a matter of fact, but Michael didn't know who they were.) I'll never forget John's generosity that night. Not six months later, on September 11, 2003, John passed away from an undetected heart condition, and the world lost a true comic genius.

The following weekend there was another Hollywood party, this time for the Oscars, but not before Michael managed to sleep over at the house. It was too soon for the boys to see him sleeping in my room, so he and I slept in a guest room and woke up early enough to sneak him into another room before the boys woke up for school. It would have felt deceptive, except for the fact that it was so important to me that I introduce Michael into their lives in the best way possible. And it had been only two and a half weeks. We were moving fast, but maybe too fast for the kids to understand. The boys were with me most of the time, not only because of Rob's unpredictable work schedule but also because Rob was gracious enough to let them really feel that this was their home. They spent all of their weekdays with me and an occasional weekend with him when he was in town. That's why integrating Michael into their house and lives had to be handled the right way. Dropping off the boys at school that morning, knowing that Michael was at home waiting for me was the first rush of feeling what my life was going to be like once we all lived together.

The next day I was going to get the opportunity to see Michael in his element at a tapas restaurant and a samba club. Having lived in Brazil for ten years, Michael spoke fluent Portuguese and Spanish and had eaten, drunk, and danced all over Mexico and South America. When he showed up at the house and Nicky was trying to ask him something, I noticed his eyes were glassy and that he was most definitely stoned. I flashed back on being in his bedroom days before, and just like the Carrie Wells character with HSAM in the TV show *Unforgettable* (who was inspired by me), I remembered that I had seen rolling papers on his desk.

This was a deal breaker for me.

I didn't know how much or how often he smoked dope, but I knew we'd discuss it the next day. Whatever the amount, I didn't want it around my seven- and eight-year-old boys. I knew Michael was wild in college. Very wild. And I'd heard enough about his former druggie experiences the first night we went out. But I had thought it was all past him now. He seemed more like someone who could knock back a few drinks and debate you, rather than someone who would light up a joint, or more, and drop out. I was never a drug person. Ever. And I really didn't see myself raising my boys with someone who got stoned just to get through.

The next day I told him how I felt and he said he smoked to relax and would never do it around me or the boys, but he couldn't see the harm. We realized that the reason we never dated in college, besides Linda and the girlfriend code, of course, was because I was way too straight for Michael. And maybe still was. Only time would tell. But in the meantime, he promised never to smoke when he knew he would see me. My plan was to see him so often, there would be no time to smoke. We were about to go away for a whole week together to Mexico for what Michael called the first of three honeymoons. We were that much in love and planning our future together. Plus there was another red carpet event for an Oscar party the day before we left. Michael could wear his new tuxedo and get his hair tjuzed out by MaryAnn for the third time. All that life, full of love and hope, and it had been only three weeks.

March 24 – May 21, 2003

There's nothing like vacation sex.

Michael and I were on fire. Out of the country, away from our daily lives, and taking each other in 24/7 was strangely comfortable for two people who had known each other for a long time, but had never shared a common space. To an outside observer, it may have looked like we were racing to get on a fast track to the rest of our lives, but to us, being together seemed effortless and easygoing. If our relationship seemed fast and furious, it was only to make up for the time we lost not being together all those years.

But I knew then what I know now: we would never be the people we are today without all those years between college and now. And I'm forever grateful that Michael hadn't come to that dinner in 1998 when Paul and Janet and Richard and Rob and I got together. If Michael had walked into the restaurant, with the way I've always felt about him and the state of my marriage at the time, it would have been a disaster that I would be dealing with to this day. He would have been the tipping point that would have broken up my marriage, and there would have been too many bodies to step over trying to get to each other. As far as I was concerned, anyway. I once asked Michael what would have happened if we had reconnected at that dinner. He looked at me and said point-blank, "I'd never sneak around with another man's wife."

But that didn't happen, thank God, and now we were just two lovers in Mexico getting to know each other and falling more in love. The hotel room at the Marquis Reforma was small, but very well appointed—beautiful dark wood cabinetry and every amenity for the traveler. I'm the type who loves to make a hotel room a home away from home. It's from all my years as an actress on location. As soon as I hit a hotel room, I hang up every item, fill every drawer, lay out all my toiletries on a towel, and take out the pictures or candle I've brought.

Michael paid no attention to the way I was setting up our room. I, on the other hand, was checking out every move he made. How he unpacked. (He didn't. Clothes left scrambled in his suitcase or draped over surfaces after use.) How he ate. (As many as seven pieces of fruit in the morning followed by coffee with cream, white toast with butter, eggs, bacon, meat, and cheese throughout the day.) How he worked out. (This one was tough because we got to work out together in the hotel gym, and although I'm a dance and Pilates girl, I know enough about weights to know that his form was terrible, and I promised myself that, in addition to regular visits to MaryAnn, as soon as we got back to LA, I would turn him onto a trainer.) God, I loved his makeover potential. Here was a diamond in the rough just waiting to be polished enough to propose. Like I had said in his birthday card, I had big plans for his body.

Mexico City was the initial stop on the First of Three Honeymoons Tour because it's one of eight cities in which BrownTrout Publishers has offices. If seeing Michael order meals and talk to locals in fluent Spanish didn't make me crazy in love enough, watching him carry on business meetings dressed in his white shirt with the sleeves rolled up drove me over the edge.

Vacation sex, indeed. *Muy caliente.*

The third morning of our getting-to-know-you vacation, after another very sexy wake up, I followed Michael in the bathroom and noticed the telltale signs of blood on the side of the toilet bowl. Knowing it wasn't mine, I thought for a minute, *Did he cut himself shaving?* And remembered, *He was only in there long enough to pee.*

I know how long he takes for everything else. It was our third day together, after all.

Curiosity got the best of me, and I'm never afraid to ask the TMI questions.

"Is everything okay? I noticed a little blood in the bathroom."

"Sometimes I have blood in my urine. I've had it for two years. It's not a big deal. I checked it out with my urologist. He said it might be from a kidney stone or a gallstone or from taking too many supplements. It's really nothing."

"What? Blood in the urine is never *nothing*. Especially over two years. And I've never heard of its coming from too many supplements. You barely take any, anyway. You have to get this checked out as soon as we're back in LA. I have great doctors you can go to. You must see my number one health doctor, Dr. Khalsa. Promise me, as soon as we're back you'll get this checked."

Michael promised and the rest of the trip we put the blood in his urine on the back burner, as we enjoyed the beautiful cities of Cuernavaca and Taxco. Two lovers who were playing for keeps and couldn't keep their hands off each other. We met people Michael had known for years, and they all couldn't believe how happy he seemed and how perfect we were as a couple. We had lunch with his friends at La Hacienda de Cortez, and touring the grounds, found ourselves at one extraordinarily beautiful spot, when Michael turned to me and said, "I know what you're thinking." I felt busted because I was thinking what he thought I was thinking. But before I could explain or protest, he said, "I know what you're thinking because I'm thinking the same thing. This would be a great place for a wedding."

We hadn't been dating a month and we were already talking about happily ever after. When you're with the right person, it's as natural as breathing. But with what I'd observed about Michael's health, I knew certain changes had to be made. Little did I know those changes would have to come a lot sooner than I expected.

Michael

When I told Marilu about the blood in the urine, she could not believe that I had let this go on for so long. I tried to convince her, repeating the nonsense that I had heard from my doctors, that everything was okay. She would have none of it. I felt foolish but still did not have the fear that I should have had.

We spent the first days of our trip in Mexico City, then took an SUV over the mountain and down to the beautiful colonial city of Cuernavaca. I had been to this city with my parents some years before, and thought Marilu might like the hotel once owned by Lauren Hutton. The city is big now, but the colonial center is beautiful and our hotel was chic and modern.

On the advice of friends we took a day trip to see the ancient city of Taxco. The long drive across the barren landscape made me remember my life of ceaseless wandering. As we climbed the hill to Taxco my mind went to my first impulse, honed for many years. I wondered what it would be like to live in this city, to leave everything behind. To start fresh. But, indeed, I was starting fresh, with Marilu next to me as we were exploring this fascinating city together. From the colonial Baroque cathedral at the top we picked a street to take down the hill and wandered through narrow, steep lanes of tropical fruits and colorful flowers, of parrots and monkeys in cages, with children playing everywhere on the crowded sidewalks.

That evening we drove back to Cuernavaca, but first we stopped at a hacienda to visit my friends who were vacationing there. An amazing place, this old monastery had been converted and was now used for weddings and corporate gatherings. These friends had known Gloria. But when they met Marilu they could see I had someone special, that she was not just another gringa. Marilu was sweet and curious and so loving with people. Emma and Rogelio vindicated my thoughts, and they confirmed what I had been feeling, that I was right about this girl.

We had such a wonderful trip, but the return to the States was terrible. A fine journey negated by some filthy peanuts bought from a street vendor. Marilu turned green while on the plane; I have never seen anyone get so sick so quickly. This incident led us to another path of my health journey, the campaign to rid myself (and Marilu) of parasites. A long and frustrating road that was!

Marilu

The whole vacation was perfect until I decided to buy some peanuts off the street in Mexico City right before we left for the airport. By the time I hit the business class lounge, I was already feeling that distinct *my body can't handle what I just ate* feeling, and, throughout the flight, I was so violently ill with food poisoning that the flight attendant told me I was the sickest passenger she'd ever seen. And this was her usual route. Of all the times she's flown, my turista was the worst. Wow. She even said, "You're green." (Elphaba green?) I knew that in addition to dealing with Michael's blood in his urine, I'd be dealing with whatever was ailing me, as well.

Besides having to do several rounds of antibiotics until we found the right combination to kill whatever I had picked up in Mexico, the next few weeks were all about integrating Michael into my boys' and my day-to-day lives. He would drive the thirty-three miles most days from his office to my house, just so we could spend the night together, and then he'd leave in the morning before the boys woke up. That is, until the morning of my birthday, when they decided to surprise me with a breakfast bowl of fruit and knocked on my bedroom door with a "Happy Birthday, Mommy!" I went out into the hallway to tell them, "Michael had a sleepover!" They loved that he was there, because by that time, he already seemed like part of the family. The four of us bonded quickly, and the boys went exploring with Michael in his Palos Verdes neighborhood like they were Tom Sawyer to his Huckleberry Finn. We played board games on Friday night and, no matter how many properties he mortgaged in Monopoly or how few triple letters he landed on in Scrabble, Michael always seemed to win. Soon he was the guy you most wanted on your team and everyone's phone-a-friend. My boys adored him, and one day Nicky said, "Mommy, when you marry Michael, and notice I said *when* and not *if*, can Joey and I give you away?" When we married on December 21, 2006, they did just that. And as part of our vows, I read a birthday card from the boys to Michael in 2004, just one year after we first got together that said, "Since you've come into our lives, you have made us so happy, and we take no shame in saying we love you." Nick, not even ten years old at the time, knew how Michael completed our family.

BESIDES THE BOYS, IN MAY of 2003 there were other family members to get to know. Michael and I both come from enormous villages of blood relatives and extended family members. Between dinners with my sister and two brothers and two nieces and their broods that live in LA, we decided to take our relationship to New York during one of Michael's business trips so that Michael could meet my sister Christal and her family, as well as see Michael's first Broadway show—*Nine* with Antonio Banderas—and hang out backstage at *Chicago* to show off my fabulous new guy.

It was a busy time of year for Michael's traveling schedule, and he kept promising me that the appointment with his urologist was forthcoming. I'd only seen blood in his urine that one day in Mexico City, but the whole thing still didn't feel right to me. I gave him until the middle of May to make an appointment; otherwise I was taking charge.

CHAPTER SIX

May 22, 2003
Marilu

By the time Michael made an appointment with the urologist who had performed his cystoscopies for the past two years and had given him an "all clear"—despite the fact that there was recurring blood in his urine—the doctor had retired and a younger doctor in the office was going to take over the case. Michael made his cystoscopy appointment for Thursday, May 22, 2003, the same day I had planned to go with my brothers Lorin and Tommy to El Paso, Texas, to close out our uncle's home. I wanted to go with Michael to his appointment, but it had taken so long for him to make one that I didn't want him to postpone it for another few weeks or so. His work schedule was so crazily busy during that time of year that who knew when he could go again? I couldn't change my plans because airline tickets were bought, and organizing the people involved in the move had taken some time. My brothers and I had to go on that day.

Besides, Michael was very reassuring that this was no big deal, even though I had an intuitive feeling otherwise. His brother Rob would be taking Michael to the appointment, which was located much closer to where they both lived. We said our goodbyes and Michael headed to the Palos Verdes area to spend the night before his appointment, and Lorin and I headed to El Paso to see Uncle.

Uncle was not only our Chicago neighborhood's art teacher, astrologist, and amateur vet, he was also the first natural food advocate and holistic health-minded person I knew, healing sick and injured stray animals from the neighborhood and giving advice about natural remedies to whoever would listen. He used products like green soap for disinfection and homemade herbal broths for nourishment. He believed in natural cures over pills and was a strong influence in my life, especially in diet and nutrition. Uncle was a real character. He and Charles had moved to El Paso in 1989 from the outskirts of Chicago to live with Charles's sister, Nina, after her husband died.

In February of 1994 Uncle had suffered a stroke. I was six months pregnant with Nicky at the time, and if I had not called Uncle during a lunch break from *Evening Shade* just to check in, I don't know what would have happened. Charles told me, "Dan hasn't moved for almost two days now. He's just lying on the floor refusing to accept help!" I immediately called an ambulance in El Paso. The doctors later told me that he had suffered a brain stem stroke and had been just a few hours away from death had he not received medical attention when he did. He survived his stroke but was never quite the same, and now, nine years later, was forced to move into a nursing home because Nina had passed away and Charles was dying of Alzheimer's disease in the same extended-care hospital. They were lucky enough to be roommates because a considerate hospital administrator recognized the bond between them and wrote them up as "cousins."

By 2003, Uncle and Charles had been together for over fifty

years, the longest and most successful relationship in our family. They became a couple a few months before I was born, but now, sadly, a half-century later, disease and time were bringing their relationship to an end. The plan was for my brothers and me to meet in El Paso to gather Uncle's remaining possessions from their house. Lorin and I drove from Los Angeles on Wednesday, May 21, to meet our brother Tommy, who was flying in from Chicago that evening.

Thursday morning I woke up full of trepidation about Michael's procedure but eager to face this adventure with my brothers. We'd first visit our uncle in the nursing home and then go off to his home to pack up his stuff. Our visit to the nursing home was very encouraging: Uncle was in fine form, funny and cute with his usual touch of cynicism. He wasn't as sharp as he had been before the stroke, but there was no reason to doubt that he would be around for several more years. After visiting Uncle, my brothers and I went to his house to organize and pack up more than fifty years of family history. We all knew there would be a lot of fascinating old photographs, cassettes, LPs, and artwork, but I was also a nervous wreck because my mind continued to stray to Michael's cystoscopy that morning.

With every phone call, he reassured me that my presence back in LA wasn't necessary because his brother Rob was there to drive and assist him. I couldn't relax, though. That little voice inside told me something was wrong. Cystoscopies rarely take more than an hour, and his was scheduled for early-morning Los Angeles time, so I expected to hear from him by noon El Paso time. When he didn't call by lunchtime, I knew something was up and grew more and more upset and worried as the day wore on. It was difficult to hold back tears.

Here I was with my two brothers, whom I've known and loved all my life, sifting through our uncle's collection of family photos, videos, scrapbooks, and souvenirs that documented our childhood, our family, and his beautiful, enduring relationship that was now coming to an end. How lucky Uncle and Charles were to have had each other as soul mates for so many years, beautiful to see as Michael and I were at the beginning of our relationship. I had finally found my soul mate, someone I loved so deeply, and his life and our relationship were in jeopardy. Would we soon be closing shop after a brief, lovely time together? My whole life, I'd wanted to have what Uncle and Charles had. They were my role models. I needed to believe that this was only the beginning of Michael's and my long journey together.

With all these emotions at play, I kept returning to my worst fears. After trying him several times, I couldn't believe that it was taking him so long to call me back. But when he finally called, the relief was brief, given his news.

His new, young doctor told him that it looked like he had bladder cancer, but not to worry too much because the bladder cancer he has is similar to skin cancer in that it grows like little skin tags that can be easily loped off. He told Michael to return in a week when the labs results would be in and he'd have more information. I said to Michael, "Did he actually use the word *cancer*?" And Michael said, "Yes, the word *cancer* did come up, but the doctor didn't seem worried." I told him that I was definitely going with him to his next appointment. I didn't want to let on how concerned I was or how many questions I had that I'm sure he never asked or that his doctor never answered. That first conversation about Michael's bladder cancer took place on the steps of Uncle's house, where the reception was bad and both Michael and I were losing

Outstanding Teenager of Illinois a few months before starting at the University of Chicago. Notice my puffy dairy nose and face.

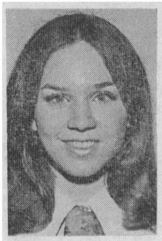

Teen Honored

Marilu Denise Henner has been named 1970 Outstanding Teen-ager of Illinois by the Outstanding Americans Foundation. She is daughter of Mrs. Joseph P. Henner and late Mr. Henner. Miss Henner is now competing with other state winners for one of two national outstanding teen-ager titles and scholarships.

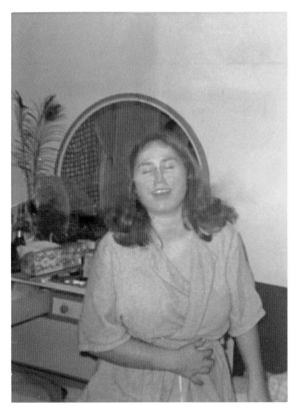

My weight at an all-time high within weeks of meeting Michael.

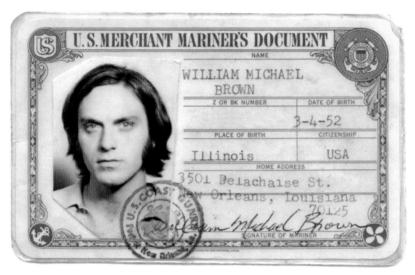

New Orleans 1974, the Seaman's Card that allowed Michael to ship
out as an *Ordinary Seaman/Wiper.*

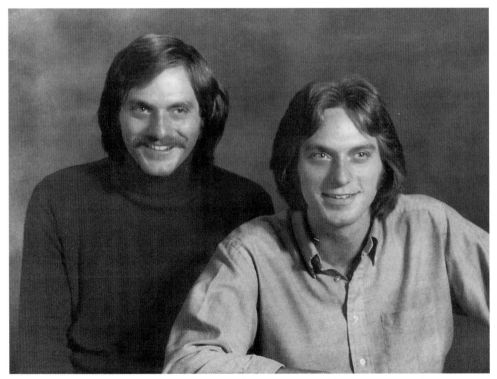

Michael back in Utah while on leave from offshore work in Brazil
with Marc, his twin brother, on the left, May 1977.

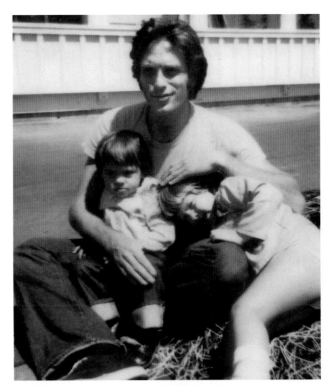

Michael with his daughters baby Cassia and Carine sitting on the dock in Port Hueneme, CA, April 1980.

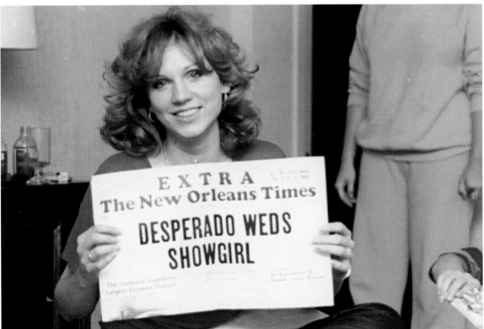

The day after running into Michael at the New Orleans Courthouse, which was the day before marrying my first husband.

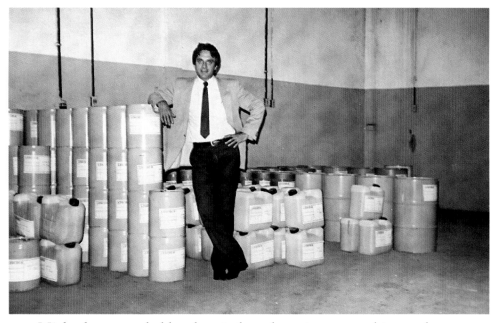

Michael surrounded by chemicals and carcinogens at his warehouse
in Rio de Janeiro, October 1988.

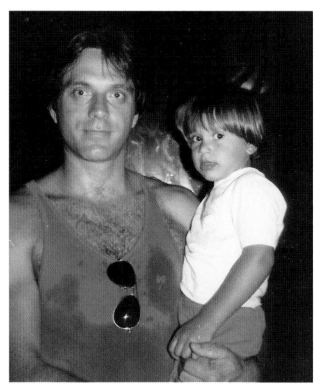

Michael holding his son,
Michael, in spring 1988.

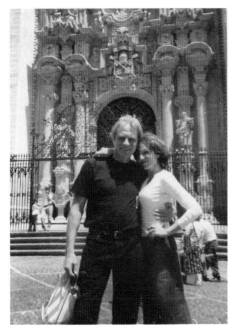
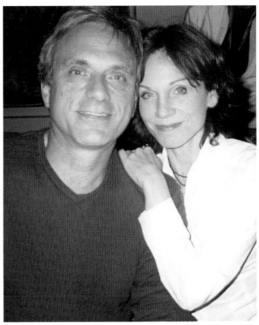

LEFT: March 2003, four weeks after our first date. Feeling madly in love in Taxco, Mexico, unaware that Michael would be diagnosed with bladder cancer two months later. RIGHT: May 4, 2003, our first trip to New York after two months of dating.

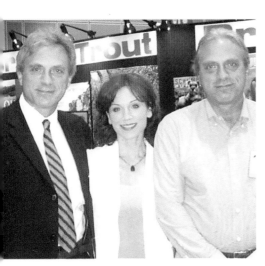
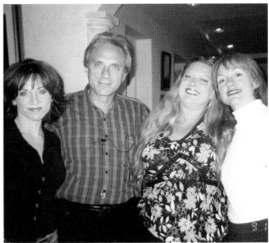

LEFT: Michael wearing a tie, me, and his twin brother, Marc, at Book Expo, May 30, 2003, the day after Michael was diagnosed with cancer. RIGHT: From left: Me, Michael, his daughter Carine, and his sister Julie, June 2003.

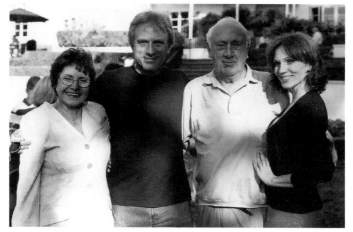

Michael and me hanging out with his parents, Bill and LaRae, in San Mateo, CA, early August 2003.

Michael's family reunion in San Mateo, CA, August 2003, the day after discovering the spot on his lung and two days after undergoing his first BCG treatment for his bladder cancer. Left to right: Julie, Jon, Michael, me, Marc, Wendover, Marc, and Rob.

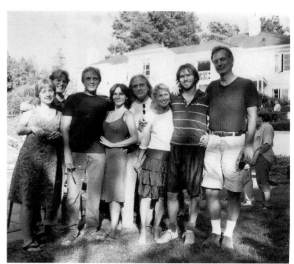

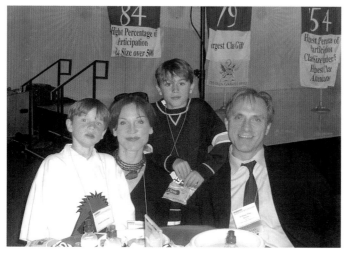

June 5, 2004, our 30th class reunion at the University of Chicago. Joey, me, Nick, and Michael. Our happy little family that weathered the storm.

Michael and me in Poggio, Italy, July 2004. On our first family trip to Europe feeling healthy and strong and more in love than ever.

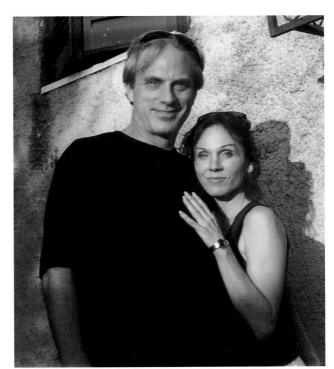

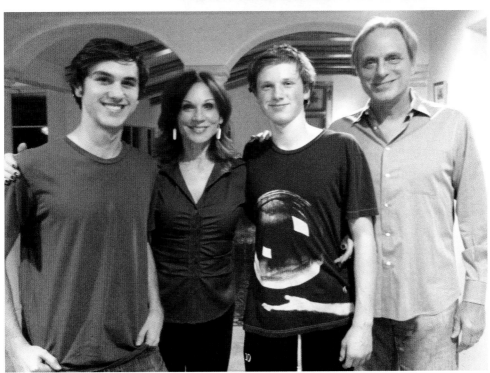

Nick, Joey, Michael, and me in 2012.
There's nothing like a healthy, happy family!

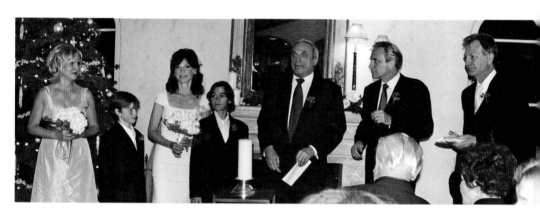

December 21, 2006, our wedding day, a true family affair. My sister
Christal, Joey, me, Nick, Marc, Michael, and Rob. The boys walked me
down the aisle and gave me away, just like Nick predicted they would.

battery. Michael's voice seemed far away and uncertain. I wanted to crawl through the phone and be with him to see how he was really feeling—and looking.

This was back in 2003 so, of course, I couldn't just pull up my iPhone and do instant research about bladder cancer. We finished packing Uncle's stuff, and I was forced to be patient and informationless about bladder cancer during the thirteen-hour drive back to LA with Lorin, which gave me plenty of time to think. What struck me the most about this experience of packing up Uncle's most important possessions was how much stuff we accumulate in our lives. We are so afraid of letting things go. It's great to have those things to reminisce and trigger great memories, which is probably the main reason we do it. But as great as those things are, they are just things. Nothing compares to the people we love. I thought about how Uncle and Charles would have gladly parted decades ago with every one of those possessions just to have one extra week together, and how much I would gladly part with everything I own to have more time with Michael.

Lorin and I sped back to LA, stopping only for gas, snacks, and bathroom breaks, because I couldn't wait to hear more about Michael's procedure and to gather as much information about bladder cancer as possible. While driving the SUV, my mind was racing with a plan. I wouldn't go only to the obvious medical sites. The first three pages of any Internet search are usually connected to someone who is paying for the privilege of being there. Very often it's a pharmaceutical company. My plan was to go to the more obscure health sites that might not have a budget, but have some of the best information. I read everything I can and, even when I find contradictions among the glut of articles, there emerges a pattern that—when I read enough varying opinions—helps me find the truth of what works for me. I'm wary of following just one point of view. Everything has to be evaluated within its own context.

There was so much to read, so much to learn. If Michael's cancer were truly no big deal, as his doctor said, then we'd still have to figure out where it came from and what he can do about it now. At this point I knew enough about health to know that Michael should immediately begin detoxing his body. Everything from skin brushing to rebounding to colonics to giving up meat, dairy, and sugar—the tenets of the *Total Health Makeover*—would become part of his daily regime. From now on everything he did would be judged by how it may be affecting his cancer. He would see all the great doctors I'd worked with over the years since my own health journey began in 1978 and listen to what everyone had to say.

The ride home to LA was fast and furious in a good way. There's nothing like a thirteen-hour road trip to help you gather your thoughts. Michael was waiting for me at the house, and I barely stopped the car before I ran into his arms and we held each other for a long time. I was more resolved than ever to live a long life with the man of my dreams, and, before we even returned the minivan, we grabbed the boys and headed to dinner at Real Food Daily for a healthy vegan meal. We'd eat macro plates with brown rice and beans, fermented foods, daikon and seaweed, at least for a while, as we figured out our next steps. He could even have a vegan Caesar salad or my special cold soba noodles. I wasn't taking away the flavor; only what I call the *health robbers*—processed foods, meat, sugar, and dairy—and replacing them with life-giving nutrient-dense foods. Since 1979 I had been saying to everyone, "Change your palate, change your life." And it was now time to put that into action and prove it to Michael.

Michael

Finally, in April 2003 my useless old urologist retired and I was given a new one. At this point, due to the urging of Marilu, I had become anxious to go to a new urologist and see what he said about this bleeding. I remembered what my general practitioner had said a couple of years before, that maybe the bleeding was caused by cancer.

Meanwhile, I went to Marilu's orthopedic doctor to check on a chronically sore right knee. The doctor was a friend of Marilu's and quite popular among the Hollywood crowd. I met with him and went through my symptoms, at which point he ordered up an MRI of my knee. The results came back as a torn meniscus. I was, therefore, scheduled for corrective surgery for the week after my cystoscopy.

My brother Rob took me that day for my first real cystoscopy. I went under with the full anesthesia, the first time in my life I had ever had an operation. When I awoke I was lying in the recovery room with several other patients and a bunch of nurses. I was vaguely aware of my surroundings, still feeling a glow from the anesthesia that I did not want to shake off. My brother came into the room and stood by my bed. You would have thought a party was going on, everyone was joking and laughing. These were my last moments of blissful ignorance. My doctor entered the room. He said to me, "We found tumors in your bladder. You have cancer." Silence fell over the room. That doctor knew how to kill a party. I was still a bit groggy and did not react except to ask what to do now. He told me to come back in a week, after the results of the biopsy were available. I looked around the room and said, "You can go back to your party now," and laid my head down. Finally I knew what was causing the blood in my urine; in some way, I felt relieved.

Though the doctor had found the tumors, the tumors had not been biopsied or *staged*. In general, the biopsy confirms the doctor's diagnosis and identifies what type of cancer is present. The staging determines where the cancer falls on the number line from stage 1 to stage 4—the higher the number, the worse, more progressed the cancer. Needless to say, the bladder cancer pushed my torn meniscus and the pending knee surgery to the back burner, as I now needed to focus entirely on the cancer.

When I heard that Marilu was coming straight back from a trip to Texas, I went to her house to meet her. I knew that I had to start doing something about this cancer, and was anticipating that Marilu would have a plan. When she and her brother Lorin got back in record time, I again felt whole as I was with my loving woman.

May 24–31, 2003
Marilu

While we waited to get back the lab results of the cystoscopy, I became obsessed with learning everything I could about bladder cancer. I knew I would be going with Michael to his follow-up appointment on May 29, and I wanted to be ready with questions. After learning that there are two types of bladder cancer, I wasn't going to let Michael take any chances. Eighty percent of the time bladder cancer presents as the papillary type that grows up like a small stalk and can be lopped off like a skin cancer tag. And the other 20 percent it presents as a CIS (carcinoma in situ), which is red, flat, and velvety, and lives on the surface, which can grow down and metastasize into other organs. As Michael's Doctor Concierge, there was no way I wasn't going to do my homework and find the best team possible. I was not going to let him down.

In addition to the follow-up appointment, the week was action-packed with getting ready for BookExpo America, the annual trade show for the publishing industry. I had attended several expos with my various books, and Michael had presented at BookExpo with a BrownTrout booth ever since 1989, but strangely enough, we had never run into each other over the years. (Once again it was obvious we were meant to reconnect exactly when we did.) This year I was doing a signing for my book *Healthy Holidays*, and Michael had his entire team in Los Angeles to man the enormous Brown-Trout booth and meet with prospective customers. BookExpo runs Thursday through Sunday, so weeks before we knew about Michael's diagnosis, we'd begun planning to throw a company party for forty people at my house that Thursday night. Michael had asked that we serve Mexican food, which I always love to serve because when you do it with brown rice and beans and guacamole and salsa, it's really healthy. But Michael had asked that, in addition to the vegan options and the fish and chicken I don't mind serving at the house, we also serve carnitas for his gang.

Now, anyone who knows me knows that in all the years I've lived in my house, I have never served beef, pork, or veal. Never. Long before the World Health Organization announced the link between red meat and cancer, declaring it carcinogenic, especially when cooked at high temperatures, I had been warning people not to eat red meat, and to absolutely avoid feeding it to their children. My boys have never eaten red meat or had a cheeseburger or a beef or pork hot dog (or had a glass of milk, for that matter), and they are healthy, strong, and tall. When friends heard that I was willing to serve barbecued meat for Michael's party, they all said, "It must really be love for you to honor his request." And all I could think of after his diagnosis was, *Enjoy your last carnitas, Mister. No more meat or dairy for you after this party!*

The party was on the same Thursday as the follow-up appointment, but the night before was also a big deal. My *Taxi* buddy Tony Danza was performing his club act at the Roosevelt Hotel, and we had arranged to go and see him, not one, but two nights that week. On Wednesday, we were taking a group of Michael's coworkers, and on Friday, we were going with my other fellow *Taxi* buddies, Danny DeVito, Jim Brooks, and Chris Lloyd and their dates. It was Michael's big introduction to a very important part of my life, and I couldn't wait to proudly show him off. We all, in fact, had dinner at the same restaurant as Michael's and my second date less than three months earlier when he and I knew that our first time was imminent. I couldn't help but think about how far we had come in such a short time; less than three months and we were already such a couple.

Seeing Tony's show on Wednesday and his meeting Michael and his gang was everything I knew it would be. Along with Jim Brooks, Tony is my closest friend from the *Taxi* days, and he has always been fun and gracious to everyone I've introduced him to. He and I have been there for each other through marriages, divorces, openings, and closings, and that night on stage at the Roosevelt Hotel nightclub he was in rare form. Michael was surprisingly festive, and he and Tony really hit it off, and, at one point, Tony turned to me and said, "Mar, he's great. He's great, Mar." He could see how happy I was in this relationship, which was not always the case. There's nothing like seeing a really good friend to take your mind off the threat of bad news. Hanging out with Tony the night before Michael's follow-up appointment was a great reminder of a long and happy life, and that, no matter what we would hear the next day, there are constants in one's life to help gauge milestones. Michael slept over again that night so that we could drop off the boys at school and I could take him to his appointment.

I woke up happy because Michael was in my home and in my bed. The boys had already spent so much time with him and felt so close to him; it all felt so right. And then I remembered that today was the day that life may change. It was a Thursday, which meant the boys' school had a family breakfast, so we all piled into Michael's car, which is a Lexus convertible sports car with a very tiny backseat. The boys were so young and small that they loved sitting back there, especially when I was willing to ride with the top down. With the feeling of wind in our faces, Joey in his little hat to block his ginger skin from the sun, and blasting music Nicky chose on the radio, I kept thinking, *I am so happy. I want to remember this always. We are a family now. And no matter what happens next, we will handle it. It's all going to be okay.*

We said goodbye to the boys and their friends after breakfast and headed down to Michael's doctor. The office could only be described as unassuming and mini-mall-medical-center sterile. Michael's doctor was not my kind of doctor, either. Rather mono-syllabic, not at all thorough, and somewhat annoyed that I was asking for specifics. When I referred to the two kinds of cancers, he kept saying things like, "It's the stalk kind that grows up, like a skin tag. I lopped it off. It's not a big deal. Come back the first week in September."

I still didn't feel resolved with his answer and asked, "So does he have cancer?"

His quote was: "He has it, but I lopped it off."

"So it's gone? Is there anything else Michael should do? Any foods he should eat or stay away from? Any other protocol he should follow?"

"Nothing else, just come back in four months."

I didn't want to alarm Michael, but I was in a blind rage. I already hated his old doctor for having missed the bladder cancer for two years, but now I hated his new doctor even more for being so blasé and not thorough in his diagnosis and explanation. I wanted to weigh my words carefully, so as not to scare Michael into going blindly with his doctor's request to just come back in a few months. I didn't want Michael to take the path of least resistance so many patients take because it seems easier to just follow their doctor's orders than to question every little thing they're being told. People often prefer to walk like lemmings over a ledge to their unquestioned fate than to do the necessary homework and risk being annoying or unpopular because they demand more information and options. But I have never been one to back off from controversy when it comes to protecting someone I love or defending a position I believe in. So when we got to the parking lot, I blurted out, "I don't trust this doctor. This does not seem right. I want you to go to my doctors, starting with Dr. Khalsa. September is way too long to wait. We're not waiting anymore for the right information." I could tell that Michael was still reeling from the news, which was totally understandable. And he had an office full of people in town whom he had to deal with. I knew, too, that his mind couldn't possibly take in all that I had to say. Not yet, anyway.

I dropped Michael off at work and drove his car back to my house to get ready for that night's party, my mind racing with our next steps. Getting Michael in to see Dr. Soram Khalsa was first on the agenda, and because of my history with Khalsa, I knew I could set up an initial consultation appointment for Michael to meet him and hear what he might recommend in terms of further tests, procedures, and supplements. Dr. Khalsa had been my primary care physician for many years at that point. He is not only a full-on American Medical Association MD, but he is also the greatest integrative medicine doctor I have ever met. A brilliant diagnostician, he is like a medical detective who is always able to figure out what a patient needs and then is able to utilize the perfect combination of Western and Eastern practices. Over the years, I have sent many people to Dr. Khalsa, and I've never seen him fail to target exactly what the person needed in terms of diagnostic measures, procedures, supplements, and the opinions of other specialists. I knew, too, that before accepting Michael as a patient, Khalsa would want Michael to write out his complete health history, explaining in as much detail as he could any past illnesses and, in his case especially, any exposures to what Khalsa calls the *total body burden* of chemicals absorbed by a person over time. This includes places you may have lived near hazardous materials or polluted soil or water, toxins you may have ingested from smoking or doing drugs, or even your sushi-eating habits, which might lead to taking in too much mercury from fish. I knew that Michael had been a party guy in college and that he had been exposed to toxic chemicals in boiler rooms and the like during his merchant seaman days. What I didn't know was to what extent the other people among his family and friends would support the changes in Michael's normal that he would be making.

Years ago I had experienced my own family's shocked reaction when, after months of nutritional research and changing my normal, I came home for Christmas in 1979 and said, "I now know what killed Mommy and Daddy! It was their lifestyle and stress and eating habits!" And they all looked at me like I was crazy when I wanted them to stop serving roast beef and Yorkshire pudding on Christmas Eve and swap it out for healthier organic fare with some vegan options. Sometimes it takes a family a while to adjust to a person's new behaviors. I have learned from my years of teaching online classes at marilu.com—a website I started in 1999 to give people who read my books even more information—that getting healthy and changing what people know as your normal is often threatening to family members who don't want to give up, or even examine, their own unhealthy habits. I was in the business of saving Michael's life, but we were less than three months into our relationship; how would the rest of his people react when Michael started even the basics of a detox program?

When I began my health journey in 1979, one of the first things I learned was the benefit of skin brushing. Every day, your body sheds about two pounds of toxins through your urine, feces, breathing, sweat, and skin sloughing. And your largest organ (I don't care who you are!) is your skin. I had already given Michael a natural bristle skin brush and taught him how to dry-body brush first thing in the morning, before a shower or workout. Just two minutes of dry brushing your entire body with long sweeping strokes toward your heart, concentrating especially on the lymphatic areas—under arms, behind the knees, inner thighs, bottoms of feet—opens your pores, sloughs off the dead skin, and stimulates the entire lymphatic system, helping you "take out the trash" through your skin. Skin brushing also helps you sweat evenly all over, giving you a glow and keeping you from the heavy concentration of underarm sweat and smell. You need much less deodorant or antiperspirant or foot powder when you skin brush. Women can skin brush everywhere except their faces and breasts, and men should brush everywhere but their faces. For years, I had suffered with terrible psoriasis on the backs of my arms and was too embarrassed to wear anything sleeveless. The one-two punch of eliminating dairy products and skin brushing every day completely cured my psoriasis, so I've been giving people natural bristle skin brushes and teaching them the benefits of skin brushing for years. It's one thing anyone can do to improve their health.

Michael was already on board with skin brushing and was, most of the time, not eating any dairy or meat, even though he had requested I serve carnitas at the BrownTrout party, which was just hours away. After calling Dr. Khalsa's office from the car to set up Michael's first appointment, I made a mental list of what else could be done immediately to improve Michael's health—more bladder cancer homework, finding a new urologist, a more committed vegan lifestyle, and getting his loved ones on board.

I soon found out how difficult that was going to be.

The BrownTrout party that night was filled with characters that had been in Michael's life, most of them for several years. I was shocked to see how many people were drinking and smoking like it was the sixties, when we didn't know any better. I was used to a theater crowd where most people are concerned with protecting their voices and would never smoke. Not only were people lighting up, but I came upon Michael's beautiful sister-in-law and business partner teaching my seven-and-a-half-year-old Joey how to light her cigarettes. Amusing, maybe, but definitely telling as to what we were up against. I walked around the party observing the behaviors of Michael's gang, trying to grasp his normal. Michael's cancer diagnosis had only been confirmed earlier that day, so I knew only a few close friends at the party knew about it. I met so many new people that night playing hostess, but whenever Michael and I were within proximity, we would give each other a reassuring hug, as if to say, *It's all going to be all right. We are going to get through this. We are together at this time for a reason.*

Michael

A week after my fateful cystoscopy, I went with Marilu to my follow-up appointment to see the doctor. He was Indian and seemed somewhat sympathetic to alternative medicine. He told us that I should wait until September and have another cystoscopy, to see if the tumors had grown back. He said that he had resected all of the tumors; that they were papillary tumors that grew like stalks in the bladder. He assured us that this cancer was slow growing, that it was early-stage, and that if the tumors had grown back by September he would just lop them off again. When we asked what else I could do in the meantime, he said that some people believed in changing their diets and lifestyles, but that this had never been proven to make any difference.

As we went out to the parking lot, Marilu said that we were not going to wait that long to do further tests. She had not waited this long to get with the love of her life to lose him to cancer! I realized she was right. I had waited two years to get properly diagnosed; I could not wait any longer to begin to fight the cancer.

On the other hand, I did not panic over this diagnosis. I went from the clinic straight to my office, where we had a large meeting with employees from around the world, as well as the buyers from our biggest customer. That night we had a big party at Marilu's house. As I drove up to the house for the party, I had an old friend with me who had just been operated on for prostate cancer, along with other friends and colleagues. I made a joke in the car that we now had something in common: we were now in the Big C Club. Boy, was I ever in the Big C Club!

What was the reason for my complacency? Did I just believe that somehow I was immune to the worst effects of this terrible disease? Was it just plain foolishness on my part? Or did I believe that somehow this was not happening to me? All I know for sure was that as the days and weeks and months dragged on, and the seriousness of my situation became ever more apparent, my mental anguish increased, and I eventually realized that I was in a fight for my life. And as that realization seeped into me, my flippant behavior at my diagnosis seemed to ring ever more hollow. What could I have been thinking?

Marilu was, of course, also worried. As she did her research, I felt like I needed to do some also. But she was ahead of me. She found my new urologist and introduced me to Dr. Khalsa. She encouraged me to begin to do the little things that help so much, like skin brushing and colon cleansing. And she made me take all of this seriously and not sink back into complacency.

During those nights, I lay awake and recalled my childhood and the silly belief that all people lived to be one hundred and that all you needed to do was subtract your age from one hundred to know how many years you had left. This had assured me as a child, so terrified of death that I could not even speak its name. But now, with cancer forcing me to think about death all of the time, I realized how I valued life. How big a difference it made to me now if I lived to be sixty-five or seventy or died in my fifties. I had gone from thinking I had thirty or more years left to thinking I would be lucky to have five more. There was just something in the way this was playing out that I knew I had something more dangerous than my doctor had said. I felt like I was on a slippery slope, where the years I had left might be filled with pain, deterioration, disability, and sickness. My children would be forced to watch their father die while they were still so young. It made me feel so sad for them. And then there was my girlfriend, soon to be my wife, Marilu. Here was a woman who had everything and was ready to give it all up for me. And all I could do was arrive on her doorstep with cancer in my body. What could I have been thinking? How could I have been so stupid, so careless?

After that return visit to the doctor, I was not foolish enough to take comfort in what he had said, because when I thought it over, I realized that it made no sense to wait months to act. I now knew I had bladder cancer, so there had to be *something* I could do about it! As I grew ever closer to Marilu and her boys, becoming a family, I also felt as if I had a pox, something terribly wrong with me that would derail everything. And I was right, of course. There was nothing normal about my condition; the cancer had not stopped because the stalks had been lopped off. The toxicity of my body created the conditions to grow tumors every day, and I was supposed to believe there was nothing I could do about it!

But I did go on about my life and tried to act like everything was under control. My daughter graduated from college, so my entire family came to Los Angeles—my parents, brother and sister-in-law, sister, and so on. Cassia had graduated from Loyola Marymount University. This was a huge accomplishment. She had dropped out of high school to have a child and then got married. Now seven years later, she was living apart from her husband, raising her daughter, and graduating from college. I was so proud. It had been a struggle, but it reinforced in me the belief that one can never give up, that there is always hope.

Because of my daughter's mother, my ex-wife, and her tendency to misbehave, I thought it best not to invite Marilu to the graduation party. Everyone asked me about Marilu, including my ex-wife. In retrospect, I should have invited her but, at the time, I felt like I just wanted to get through this event. This gathering of my extended family was one of the first times that I revealed my new lifestyle in terms of my diet, and my father made fun of me. I think in his mind he knew that the cancer was serious, but he did not want to admit it to himself, and when he was with me and I looked okay, he must have thought the cancer might not be that bad. The rest of the family simply avoided the subject, and I did not blame them.

But it was strange not to have Marilu at the reception. She already knew all of my children so well. My girls had been very receptive to Marilu entering my life, and I was thankful for their support. Marilu was sweet and understanding with them, and it helped to break down the barriers. As I began to know the extent of my illness, I was ever more grateful that I had the support of Marilu and my daughters, because so many changes were on the horizon.

CHAPTER SEVEN

June–July 2003

Michael

As the weeks passed from the day of my diagnosis, Marilu and I became more determined to find another urologist and also an internist to help me turn my life around. Marilu is very plugged into the medical community. As a writer of books on health, and as a celebrity actress, she has access to the best doctors and healers in the world. With her help, I was able to break out of the circle of medical malpractitioners who had treated me up to this point and find people who had open minds and healing hands. She found me a new urologist, Dr. Sharron Mee, who allowed intuition to be part of her diagnostic technique. This new urologist looked at my charts and agreed with my previous doctor that I could go awhile without another cystoscopy. But we insisted that I get another cystoscopy as soon as possible. Somehow we realized that the previous doctor had not been as thorough as he should have been. Dr. Mee sensed that we were onto something and agreed to do an examination quickly, but still we had to wait six weeks after my cystoscopy of May 22 before I could undergo anesthesia again.

In early June I took a trip with Marilu and her brother Lorin to

Costa Rica to visit an organic sugar plantation. I was in a haze at this point with the diagnosis fresh in my mind and my health still at a very precarious stage. We got to San Jose and found our driver. I spoke to the driver in Spanish the entire two-hour trip while driving through the city streets and out through the countryside. As we got closer to the plantation, we could see a volcano looming in the distance. We arrived at a hotel that seemed to exist only for the plantation's guests. As we drove up the dirt road to the hotel we saw a fair-skinned man doggedly jogging along the path in the tropical heat. I turned to Marilu and said, "Only mad dogs and Englishmen go out in the midday sun."

We got to the hotel and met our hostess, Pauline, an Irish lady, who asked us if we had seen her English husband, Nigel, taking his run up the road. Indeed we had, and I shot a knowing glance at Marilu. We settled into our room and made love in the sultry heat. The walls were thin and it was easy to hear our neighbors trying to do the same thing we were doing. But it felt good being away; I felt like I could escape the cancer.

I realized during this trip how different Marilu and I had become over the many years since the University of Chicago. I had lived in Brazil for ten years, my first wife was Brazilian, and my children had been raised bilingual, English and Portuguese. I was very much at home anywhere in Latin America. Costa Rica seemed so familiar to me, but not for Marilu, who had lived in America all those years. But despite her success and fast-paced lifestyle, she was still the Marilu I knew back in Hyde Park, the girl from Chicago who wanted to dance and sing all of the time. Now I could see first-hand her love of family, her openness, her affection.

It was hard to relax, even in this beautiful setting, when I'd realize with panic that I should be getting some treatment, any treatment! I kept wondering what I could be doing to increase my chances of survival. Would I start to piss blood again? If I did, what would that mean? Was the cancer growing inside me even while I tried to change my diet and get the stress out of my life? Was it possible to destress while worrying about an active cancer growing inside your bladder? These thoughts were the constant backdrop for my trip as Marilu and I fell deeper in love.

Without Marilu, I would have lost my sanity. What was so reassuring was that she had accepted me for the poor cancer-ridden fool I was when I arrived on her doorstep. She did not step back in horror as some told her to do. She never hesitated, even though she knew the risk that I could be surgically mutilated or even die.

We took a tour of the sugar plantation. I was struck by the fact that this huge plantation, hundreds of acres of cultivated sugar cane, had only a few acres of organic sugar. The contrast illustrated what the world is up against to truly change the way people eat and the way agriculture raises food. We saw the workers wielding machetes, hauling the sugarcane out on wagons pulled by ancient tractors. And all the time I wondered, *What am I doing and why?* I kept thinking that I needed to face my disease, not run from it. Yet there I was wandering around, acting like an ecotourist. But still I tried to relax and enjoy the trip.

It was ironic that we had gone to a sugar plantation, as sugar is one thing that cancer patients must avoid. Sugar feeds the tumors, and especially refined, granulated sugar, even if it is organic. The sugar also tends to make the body more acidic, to neutralize the body's natural alkalinity. Tumors cannot grow in an alkaline environment, so returning the body to its natural alkaline state can treat and prevent cancer.

I came back from Costa Rica and had my first appointment with my new internist, Dr. Soram Khalsa. Dr. Khalsa, I learned from Marilu, is an internist from Cedars-Sinai who has a private practice in Beverly Hills. Khalsa is from Cleveland, but converted to Sikhism as a young man. He practices a combination he calls "the best of East and West." The medical technology of the West has resulted in the greatest diagnostic tools available. Unfortunately, with this diagnostic power has not come wisdom. It seems like the more precisely a doctor can diagnose an illness, the less he can prescribe a cure. Western medicine has literally gotten lost among the noise of symptoms, the clutter of test results, and the temptations of capitalist medicine, so that it cannot find the path to healing. This idea that we are going to turn off one gene to stop a disease or create some miracle drug that will go into the bloodstream and zap all of the errant cancer cells is wishful thinking and helps the patient and the doctor avoid considering the cause of the cancer and the possible natural cure. In contrast, Dr. Khalsa takes the diagnostic tools of the West and then relates their findings to the body as a whole. He seeks to strengthen the body's own defense mechanisms, to encourage the body's immune system to ward off disease. This natural way of healing, aided by modern medicine, allows him to move a patient toward health, and, as he does, the body can then heal itself.

I immediately saw the logic in Dr. Khalsa's methods. I was used to problem solving, and understanding the entire system before suggesting changes or improvements has always made sense to me. Dr. Khalsa (and Marilu, of course) had done the research. They had thought about how a person's actions impact their body and their health, from their diet, to their personal hygiene, to how they discharge waste. And Dr. Khalsa truly enlightened me to the way that all of the bodily functions working together can greatly strengthen the immune system, which is key to treating a cancer, any cancer.

Dr. Khalsa began with an exhaustive diagnosis of my body and my lifestyle. He tested my blood, my urine, and my stool. He muscle-tested me to determine my level of stress and the state of my adrenals. He hooked me up to a machine and checked my vital organs for toxic stress. He then looked at the parts and related them to the whole. When he challenged me to write an autobiography that focused on my toxic exposure, I began with my childhood, my mother convinced by doctors not to breast-feed, but rather to give me formula since I was a twin and she would never be able to handle breast-feeding us both. With her doctor's approval, my mother smoked right through her pregnancy. Raised in Utah as a young man, listening to radio reports of fallout clouds wafting over the city from the nearby nuclear test grounds of Nevada, I was told to stay indoors on certain days to avoid the worst effects of the radiation. Living near the polluted Jordan River, I—along with the other kids—chased the pesticide-spraying trucks spewing out their DDT to keep down the mosquitoes. Working in my teen years at a nursery, where I used formaldehyde to clean planter boxes until I got sick from chemical poisoning. Riding in the car with the windows rolled up while both of my parents smoked in the front seat. My own smoking habit beginning when I was only fifteen. Working in the engine room at sea, breathing benzene and diesel fumes. Working with chlorine and ethylene. Living in the pollution of New Orleans, Chicago, Los Angeles, and Rio de Janeiro. How could my poor body not become a toxic waste dump?

Dr. Khalsa diagnosed me as the most stressed-out, intoxicated patient he had ever seen. But my stress was not only chemical related. The stress of a failed marriage, children out of control, parents out of control, and business partners out of control all affected me deeply. Maybe I kept things in; maybe I made things worse for myself. But the worst part was that I did not know how to change my behavior. With this health crisis I was finally going to have to learn or die because my normal was killing me.

Marilu

The month of June was spent getting the core of Michael's medical team in place. His first meeting with Dr. Khalsa was everything I'd hoped it would be: Khalsa determining how serious Michael would be as a patient and Michael's willingness to do whatever it took to save his life. When I commented on what a good patient he was turning out to be, he knowingly explained, "Listens to and follows directions."

"What does that mean?" I asked.

"'Listens to and follows directions' is the box my first-grade teacher checked on my report card. She gave me a check plus, in fact," he said with pride. This from a seventies radical contrarian who loves bucking the status quo and challenges everything. I knew he was getting on board with this whole new way of living his life when he was eating my kale, arugula, and spinach salad on a regular basis and eschewing alcohol almost entirely.

On June 3, 2003, less than a week after Michael's urologist insisted, "Come back in September," we were in the offices of another urologist, Dr. Sharron Mee, who had been recommended by my BFF and favorite hypochondriac (and psychic-lover) Sharon Feldstein. Dr. Mee was a blond bombshell with colorful clothes and a take-no-prisoners, Erin Brockovich attitude. She recommended the immunotherapy BCG and was surprised that we were insisting on another cystoscopy so soon after Michael's recent one. She explained that we might not get a legitimate reading since the area of resection—the "I lopped it off" part—would still be inflamed. She wanted to wait at least six weeks to go back in there, which seemed reasonable enough, except that I wanted answers as soon as possible. But Michael's travel schedule during that time was already packed, so it made it easier to wait out the time for answers.

Michael's business takes him all over the world, so not only was Japan on the calendar, but he and I had two trips of our own booked—one to Costa Rica and another to Europe at the beginning of July when Rob was taking the boys on a vacation. The cystoscopy was set for July 24 with the hope that Michael's doctor was right, and that CIS would not be present. Regardless of the outcome, Dr. Mee advised that BCG treatments, once a week for six weeks, would commence immediately after the cystoscopy and that six rounds of BCG would probably be enough to take care of all of it. I was hopefully optimistic, but the more I read about bladder cancer, the more I felt Michael's doctor had misdiagnosed the big picture.

Days after meeting Dr. Mee, we were off to the Sucanat plantation in Costa Rica, which couldn't have been more exotic and romantic. Pauline McGee of Wholesome Sweeteners had invited me after seeing me on *The View* demonstrating Thanksgiving recipes using Sucanat, an acronym of *su*gar *ca*ne *nat*ural. It's from the sugarcane plant, but it is completely organic with only crushing, heating, and drying as processes (as opposed to most refined sugars, which go through several processes including being bleached, cooked in cow bones, and stripped of 90 percent of any nutrients they may have). Sucanat is also healthier than even brown sugar, which is just sugar with a dye job. Sucanat is definitely used for what I like to call *pleasure food* like desserts, but you end up using less of it because it tastes like a real food, rather than the sickeningly sweet chemical-like flavor of sugar. I first discovered Sucanat in 1985 when I was looking for an all-organic sugar for dessert recipes, and at the time, it was the easiest and healthiest sweetener for recipes that called for sugar.

It seemed strange going so far away while we waited for Michael's next results, but with Khalsa and now Dr. Mee on board I felt we were on the right path. Besides, when I asked Dr. Mee about whether or not we should go on vacation, she stopped what she was doing, looked at me seriously, and said, "Don't cancel your trips. You two should be going away when you can. You don't know the future." I knew she meant anything could happen with Michael's health, so seize the opportunity to travel when you can. But I was feeling so sure that with the right information and protocol, Michael would not only be okay, he'd be better than ever.

Costa Rica was everything that we expected and more. We completely bonded with our hosts and were impressed with the tour of the Sucanat plantation, with its simple and organic farming. Every meal we ate was vegan and another example of clean, fresh organic ingredients beautifully prepared in a simple way. As I've said for years, "Learn to love the food that loves you." And this food loved us. And, more important, Michael was falling in love with the food and the whole idea of no meat and no dairy. We walked through the hills near our hotel, talking about how to figure out a plan of action, brainstorming about what he had to prepare for his health history, and talking about marriage and what it means to be truly committed to someone even in the face of adversity. Walking through fire, as it were. And how so many couples we knew were either breaking up or having affairs to get through it all. We were so new to each other and had been through so much with other people that we couldn't pretend that relationships weren't difficult, and we promised concerted effort and open communication at all times. To this day, Michael and I refer to that walk in Costa Rica as one that solidified our commitment to each other. *In sickness and in health* is not where most people start a relationship, but we were both honest about what we were getting into and embraced the challenge.

After Costa Rica, Michael was off to Japan for work, and I was busy getting the boys ready for a summer camp near the house and shooting the Pilates DVD to go with my Body Victory kit. I couldn't believe how much had happened since the Body Victory shoot in San Francisco just three months earlier. For years I tried to do a health program as an infomercial, but I was told over and over again, "Nobody wants health." After years of begging and trying to prove to Bill Guthy and Greg Rinker that health was the new frontier, they finally took a chance and allowed me to develop a twenty-one-day program based on *The 30-Day Total Health Makeover* book. They were still worried that nobody wanted health, so there was a lot riding on the early test results for this Body Victory infomercial. But it wasn't only an eating program with recipes; the package was also to contain motivational tapes and the Pilates video I was shooting that week. Since my first class on Thursday, January 4, 1979, Pilates has been my favorite form of exercise. Whether I was getting in shape for some project or warming up before a performance of *Chicago* on Broadway or *Annie Get Your Gun* on the road, the only way I could warm up both my body *and* my voice was to do a Pilates mat workout. This was the routine I was including in the package and shooting this week. It still strikes me as ironic to be told "Nobody wants health" when I was trying to save Michael's life *with* health at the same time.

Michael's second visit with Khalsa was two and a half hours long and he discussed the personal health history that we wrote about in his health manifesto. Dr. Khalsa also thoroughly examined him and muscle-tested him for supplements. Now that's the kind of thorough doctor I was used to! At the end of it, Khalsa asked Michael what he did for a living. When Michael answered, "I'm a publisher." Khalsa said, "No. You're a cancer patient. Are you here to survive for five years? Or are you here to live a long and healthy life?" I knew what Khalsa meant. It's not enough to put your cancer in remission for five years, only to have it recur because you not only didn't change your normal, but you'd also compromised your immune system to the point where it couldn't fight off anything.

After his long meeting with Khalsa, Michael and I had a flight to catch later that day to London, where we were traveling to Europe for the first time together and meeting many of his friends and co-workers. Full of excitement, we knew it would be the same kind of sexy, intimate trip Costa Rica had been, but this time Michael was armed with more information, a better plan, and a ton of supplements. We were taking control.

Michael

I thought I knew what I was battling—bladder cancer—and that it was a relatively clean fight. Thankfully, the cancer was contained in my bladder and had not spread. There was a proven treatment, the immunotherapy known as BCG that afforded me a decent chance of beating the cancer. I was relatively young and strong compared to most men who get this disease.

When Dr. Khalsa told me during one of my initial examinations that if I wanted to survive this thing, I needed to take it seriously and make my life's work be about beating it, I thought he was being a bit melodramatic. I still retained some of the bravado that I had had when first diagnosed. The severity of my situation had not sunk in. I thought I was special, that somehow I would escape this disease without losing part of my body. I was glad I did not have prostate cancer, the cancer that all my friends seemed to get, but how did I know that bladder cancer was any better? There was no point in choosing between cancers.

A powerful technique Dr. Khalsa taught me was visualization, something I had heard about before in other contexts but only saw clearly as an option now. I learned that there are two parts to visualization for the cancer patient. As difficult and unnerving as it may be, it helps to try to understand where your cancer came from. Each cancer is unique to the person who has grown those errant cells. No two cancers are alike; they are like snowflakes. Cancer grows out of one's body, and if one is not willing to accept the cancer as a part of one's self, then that person is doomed. So attempt to accept that the cancer grows out of you. This acceptance can mature into love that enhances your appreciation for your body and your life. The cancer is a manifestation of imbalances that must be corrected if you are to survive. Visualization, which is a form of meditation, allows you to go deep into the body and *see* the cancer and from where it came. This process is continual, in that, once started, the visualization can come during a prolonged silent meditation or sporadically as you dwell on other things during the day. Once you have seen the cancer, it no longer seems so frightening.

Seeing where it came from allows you to see the path to the cure. The second part of visualization is imagining or seeing the cure: visualizing the tumors drying up and the healthy tissue returning. This visualization has healing powers, as it orients the body in a positive way and helps to relieve stress and anxiety.

This was all well and good. But, as I saw when I tried to modify my diet a few years previous, change can be difficult for family and friends. As I altered my lifestyle my cruel father noticed that I did not drink like I had before; I did not pig out on barbecued pork ribs. He would often say to me, "You may not live to be a hundred, but it will seem like you lived to be a hundred." He thought that my life would drag by as I gave up all of the small pleasures that gave his life meaning, that made it go by quickly. No more meat, no more cheese, no more strong alcohol. No more smoking dope, no more gluttonous orgies of eating burnt flesh. To be faced with so many lifestyle changes and to also have to listen to the world belittle you, that is something most healthy people do not imagine when they think of serious illness. The desire to return to normal in your life, to leave the illness behind and act like it never happened, becomes the overriding concern of most people. And if you are trying to return to normal, the world treats you with sympathy and respect. But if you try to change your life to save yourself—to move forward instead of backward—the world treats you like a traitor.

On the other hand, I was now entering a lifestyle where people were trying to heal me and themselves. There were so many positive messages, so many kind and gracious people, that it overwhelmed the negativity I felt from others. And then there were the positive effects of the changes. How much better did I feel, did I look! How quickly my body responded to the good treatment it was getting. There was no going back, as I now could feel my body strengthening each day.

Marilu was used to the awkwardness one feels when people are so concerned to find the right food for the vegans, the food "that you can eat." It is so odd that the implications of food choices, none of which have anything to do with health and nutrition, are so important to most people. But nutrition, which would seem to be the point of eating, is hardly thought of at all. Not eating meat does not mean I can't sit at the table with meat eaters or barbecue a chicken at my house. It is way too complicated to try to talk people into eating any way other than what they want at that moment. Any other thoughts contradict their need to have what they want when they want it. So people must want to change, and that usually only happens when someone gets a wake-up call, like a stroke or cancer.

There is an entire industry dependent on people trying to get back to normal. Artificial hips and knees, elbow surgeries, hair implants. Most doctors have a stake in the status quo; their jobs, or so it seems to me, are to return the patient to their normal lifestyle. How many times do we see commercials on television where the emphasis is on getting back to your job, to your life, to the golf course as the ultimate goal of cancer treatment? The doctors just don't believe that their patients are strong enough, or motivated enough, to change their behaviors, so they dumb down their "cures" and thereby condemn their patients. Add to this the fact that doctors are generally so ignorant about nutrition, it can make one wonder what inspires them to go into medicine in the first place. What can be more obvious than the fact that food is the most important contributor to health or illness?

Hippocrates said: "Let your food be your medicine and your

medicine be your food." Marilu says, "Learn to love the food that loves you." I learned from Marilu's books that food is what you take into your body every day; it is the building block of your body and thus your life. As I thought more and more about my diet, I realized that I had been poisoning myself for years. On airplanes I went from ginger ale, to cranberry juice, to water with no ice. The longer I went without sweetened or salty food, without meat or fatty milk, the cleaner my taste buds became. I was able to taste my food, and with that came a big change. I was able to finally free myself from the salty-then-sweet pendulum and go for nutrition. And how grateful my body was for this relief!

I learned from Marilu's book *Total Health Makeover* that if food is contaminated with chemicals or pesticides then those pollutants go into your body. If the food is dead meat, killed under harsh conditions, then that dead meat will bring death to your body. The larger the fish, the more mercury, as the bigger fish eat the smaller fish, and thus concentrates the mercury in its body. Likewise with animals. If we eat cows then we concentrate all of the pollution found in the cow in our bodies. The same is true of dairy products. The more concentrated the dairy product, the worse it is for the human body. Butter is worse than milk, cheese is worse than butter. How can anyone believe that curdled and aged milk can be good for anyone? How did we reach this point of disconnect with our bodies? If the food is alive, like green vegetables, sprouts, seeds, then that food gives life. There is nothing in a meat diet that cannot be found in a better and more pure form in plants. Think: in the same way that a child recoils from the smell of alcohol and finds it disgusting, the child also recoils from the putrid smell of "quality" cheese. The child knows better; the adult has grown ignorant.

By learning how to eat properly I stopped poisoning myself on a daily basis. And it did not take long for the benefits to appear. Despite the strain my body was going through dealing with an active tumor, I was actually getting stronger. As I learned to make my food my medicine, my food began to nourish me in a way that it had not ever before. (Remember, I was never breast-fed.) The net effect was much larger than simply cutting out a bad habit; I had substituted a bad behavior with a good behavior.

Detoxification is a normal bodily function that is also practically ignored by the medical community. Like a well-designed engine, many of the major systems of the body are there to carry away waste material that in our industrial age includes dangerous chemical residues and heavy metals that should not be left in the body. A Ferrari with a rag stuck in the tailpipe will not go far. The circulatory system, the urinary system, the lymphatic system, the pulmonary system, and the digestive system are all involved with waste management and discharge. If any of these systems is disrupted or does not work optimally, then the entire organism is endangered. Yet how much time is spent by the average physician, and by the average patient, on unclogging these systems? They are preoccupied with what goes in the body, but pay no attention to what comes out (or does not come out). A doctor will prescribe stool softeners and laxatives to a person with constipation but will react in horror to the idea of a colon cleansing that addresses the problem directly.

The ancient Romans were very much aware of the healthful benefits of keeping the colon clean, and in the United States colon cleansing was considered an essential part of healthcare through the 1930s. But somewhere along the line, with the encouragement and connivance of pharmaceutical companies and doctors, consti-

pation became a condition to treat with drugs. Similarly, indigestion is treated with pills, rather than looking for the cause of the
indigestion, which almost invariably is food related.

As a full-time cancer patient, I realized that detox is the one
sure way to address what "caused" the cancer—no one ever gets
to know for sure what exactly caused his or her individual cancer.
The truth is that many different things caused my cancer, though
there may be one specific activity that can be singled out as the
main culprit. Mine was smoking. Bladder cancer was smoking related. But how can that be? Lung cancer and cigarette smoking are
linked in an obvious way, since you pull the smoke through your
lungs as you breathe. But bladder cancer? Using visualization, I was
able to ponder how the smoking impacted my bladder. It is a long
way from the lungs to the bladder. But smoking is dehydrating,
which is one reason it is so bad for the skin. When the body has
less water, it produces less urine. Visualizing this process, I saw
that the contaminants from the cigarettes are flushed through the
body (leaving traces of tar and other pollutants along the way) and
end up in the bladder, mixed with the urine. This toxic brew then
sits in the bladder waiting to be discharged. I know this was true
because I smelled the toxins in my urine as I began to detox. They
smelled metallic from the heavy metals such as lead and mercury
that I had in my bloodstream. The worse the contamination, the
worse the smell. As I poured gallons of water through my system I
felt the tissue begin to clean. The return to a responsive suppleness
made me feel younger and less brittle. How could I not be encouraged by all this? And why would I not continue my health journey,
especially because I got to take this journey with Marilu?

Dr. Khalsa recommended that I get an ultraviolet sauna to help
detox out the fat cells that hold the toxins, because fat is a poison

carrier. I placed the sauna in my garage, and it was big enough for my brother Rob and me to sit in it. It was a real sauna made out of wood, but using light to heat up the body instead of heating the air to heat up the body.

One day I was having a sauna when the doorbell rang. As I got out of the sauna I saw my ex-girlfriend Gloria down at the garage door, and she was very worried about me. She had heard about the diagnosis and was there to make sure I was okay. It was a strange encounter as I was now embarked on a whole other life, yet how close the past life seemed.

CHAPTER EIGHT

Michael

By July, I was anxious to learn about my cancer but, compared to just a month prior, I was already doing much more to help myself. I was drinking large amounts of water. I was skin brushing, allowing my skin to breathe and detox. Using the rebounder to stimulate my white blood cells and to activate the lymphatic system, injecting iscador every other day, and doing colonics. Each action both helped me physically and boosted my confidence.

Our young and fresh love was still in the air. Since I had to wait to get a cystoscopy for some weeks, I decided that I wanted to take Marilu to see my office in England and to visit my agents in Scandinavia. Marilu and I flew to London in early July. I was anxious that maybe I should be doing something other than vacationing in Europe, that maybe I should be doing some treatment or other, but the new urologist, Dr. Mee, had assured me that I could wait from late May until mid-July before another cystoscopy, so I went along with my previous travel plans. Despite Dr. Mee telling Marilu, "Now is the time to enjoy something like a trip to Europe . . . who knows how many more trips you can take?"—which Marilu told me one day while teasing me—she had faith that I could beat this disease, even though no one else seemed to. There was another reason why she told me something so terrifying: to keep me on point and moving away from my previous normal existence. Her father taught her that people should be blamed for their sicknesses, not pitied, and she knew that, in many ways, I had brought on this cancer with my toxic habits. And so it was up to me to reverse this disease by moving away from the behaviors that had resulted in advanced cancer in my bladder.

At this time, so early in our relationship, I was still trying to impress Marilu—to show her that I was successful and could keep up with her. To that end, I had booked rooms at the Savoy Hotel in London. I wanted to treat Marilu in the manner to which she was accustomed, as I had promised to on one of our first dates. She had been at the Savoy years before, and so I thought we should go back there as a couple.

As soon as we arrived in London, we went straight to the hotel. Marilu did not like the first room we were given, and so, late at night, the bellman moved us to another. In my previous life, I would never have insisted on changing a hotel room, but Marilu is not one to just accept the status quo without question. Unlike me, she's always ready to advocate for her position, and in the most charming way possible (at least most of the time), which made her an effective caregiver as we navigated the complexities of the healthcare system.

The next day we walked on the Strand and hung out in Covent Garden. I tried to act natural, to avoid thoughts of self-doubt and panic, but it was difficult. After two years of failed examinations I finally knew the cause of blood in my urine, but I was not doing anything about it except taking a vacation! And I had just been in Costa Rica! It seemed bizarre and surreal.

But on the other hand, I was with Marilu and our relationship was really good. I was just then learning how to eat like a vegan. In England this can be difficult, but we found a place called Food for Thought, which was one of my first regular vegan spots. I loved the food and the atmosphere. It was a communal table arrangement with all sorts of breads and soups and many hearty meals. The more I ate this food, and the longer I went without dairy and meat, the stronger I became. Even in England, we could eat the way I needed to eat, the way Marilu had eaten for so many years. I soon became used to ordering salads in hotels, veggie dogs at Pink's, and penne arrabbiata (but no cheese)! Quite a transformation in eating habits.

After flying from London to Copenhagen, we stayed in an old-style hotel in the center of the city. I had been in Copenhagen many times when I had worked for a Norwegian ship supply company. We had a wonderful time walking the streets of the old city and spending the evening at Tivoli Gardens. My partner from England, Jack, and his wife, Gail, met us in Denmark. We went to Gothenburg, Sweden, and then on to Oslo, Norway. Walking the streets of Oslo at night took me back twenty years to my days as a shipping executive based in Rio de Janeiro. So much had changed—and was about to change—in my life.

We flew back to the U.S. and I finally moved on to the next step of my cancer journey, the first cystoscopy with my new urologist. This time I went with Marilu to Cedars-Sinai and checked in at some ungodly hour in the morning. Marilu and I were so tight by then, a true couple. These four months we'd been together had gone so fast, and while much had changed in my lifestyle, my campaign against the cancer had not even really begun. Marilu held my hand as they administered the anesthetic and I soon faded into oblivion.

As I lay groggy in the recovery room I again was surprised with the results of the examination. Not only did I have bladder cancer with the stalk-like papillary tumors, but I also had carcinoma in situ, which means *cancer on the site*. In the case of bladder cancer it is a more rare and dangerous version of the disease. It is harder to detect than the papillary tumor type, and perhaps for that reason, the other doctor missed it. It is considered much more aggressive and dangerous. The pathologist also staged my cancer, which means he calibrated the stage of advancement it had made. It was between stages 2 and 3, an advanced stage but apparently a cancer that was still contained in my bladder, one that had not invaded the muscle walls or metastasized outside the bladder. The staging was a bit speculative because there was really no way to know if the cancer was contained in the bladder or not. With the stage of my cancer set I realized how far I had let this cancer go before I did anything. I was near to stage 4 bladder cancer, which is almost invariably treated with removal of the bladder and the prostate, followed by chemotherapy. The conclusion: I was in big trouble!

For new cancer patients to learn the vocabulary of their disease is a process fraught with anxiety and panic. The patient is faced with a diagnosis that is scary enough, but added to that, he probably has no clue what the doctor is talking about. Squamous cell? Non-small cell? CIS? Or a CT scan versus CAT scan versus MRI? How exactly does metastasis work? How does the cancer spread? Is it like a virus, like a growth, like an infection? How does a cancer kill a patient? Is it a slow rot from the inside, or a catastrophic collapse of the organs? How does it feel? Does it hurt? How do I know when the end is near? Can pain be my guide? Or am I left to the mercy of the doctor, who may or may not know what to do, or care?

The patient, sick and scared, must also learn a new vocabulary. Being forced to learn this dreaded language of acronyms, obscure Latin, doctors' names, protocols, procedures, regimens—along with the resections, dissections, surgeries, cystoscopies, biopsies, blood tests, urine tests—is a frightful task. A strange combination of high school chemistry and nuclear science is used to treat cancer. No one has all of the answers. Being lost in the Tower of Babel, which is what a modern hospital is, is a big part of the experience of being a new cancer patient. No one wants to follow you down this corridor toward the cancer ward, the chronic disease future, the death row where they speak in weird tongues. And yet, there you are—alone with your fears and worst thoughts, unable to pick up the jargon quickly enough to save yourself.

Or so it felt. But I had Marilu in my corner. I could look in her eyes, hold her hand, and know that everything would come out okay. She had told me that we would make this work, and we would, even if it came down to the part with the pump! She would learn what I could not, she would ask the questions I did not, she would find a way where I might get lost. Knowing I was not alone was such a blessing. If I had not made that call in February, if I had not been ready to make a commitment, if I had gotten diagnosed before I had found my way to Marilu, then I would have been in this predicament alone. The easy answers would have then seemed more attractive, the return to normal more soothing, and I would have been lost forever.

Even though Marilu was with me every step of the way, it did not mean I went without moments of doubt and pain. I wanted so much to be strong for her, to not complain, to not make it more dif-

ficult for her. This was silly, as our love was too great at this point
to be weighed down by disease. She wanted to be there for me, so
I had to learn to let her all the way in. When she told me that we
would make it work, no matter how mutilated I might become, I
knew her love was there for me. But still it took me months to listen
to my heart and allow myself to give in all the way.

With the results of this cystoscopy in hand, we consulted with
Dr. Mee on a course of treatment. The standard treatment for
bladder cancer, BCG, which is known as an immunotherapy, has
been used for more than thirty years to treat superficial bladder
cancer with great success. Immunotherapies are not chemotherapies, though many times laymen discuss them as if they are the
same thing. Chemotherapy is given to cancer patients as a systemic
treatment to stop the spread of cancer in the body while also treating specific tumors. Chemotherapies are chemicals that have been
shown to be effective in killing cancer cells in tumors and that
are traveling in the body through the blood or lymphatic systems.
Immunotherapies, on the other hand, are treatments designed to
imitate a viral attack on an organ, thereby stimulating the immune
system to attack the virus and by extension to attack the cancer
cells in that organ. BCG is a form of bovine tuberculosis; by injecting it into the bladder, the immune system focuses its attention on
the bladder and in theory destroys the cancer cells.

Marilu

There is a routine you get into when hanging out in a hospital
waiting room. You can tell the newbies with their summer clothes
and lack of sweaters, books, comfort food from home, and phone

chargers. We veterans always come prepared for the long haul because we've learned the hard way that there's nothing worse than a protracted stay in a waiting room without the usual creature comforts and necessary supplies. You can spot the different combinations of families as they homestead around the room while waiting for postoperative news from their respective doctors. Each time the door marked *Hospital Staff Only* opens, you can feel the collective gasp as the various family groupings freeze, holding their breaths for a second, thinking, *Whose doctor is this? What are they saying? Is it good news?*

The news is always obvious, even when you can't hear what the doctor has said to the alpha person in each group. Over my years of observing waiting room results, I've seen people do everything from applauding to screaming to fainting to flailing. I remember when my father died from an acute heart attack during a Christmas party in our home, my mother and I rode in the ambulance to the hospital, but I knew he was already gone. We pulled into the emergency entrance, where they rushed him in and worked on him for a few minutes before coming out to tell us, "I'm sorry, that's all we can do." The moment was surreal. When my two older sisters arrived, one of them broke down and the other one smashed her hand up against the wall with such force that she almost needed stitches. You never know how people will react to hearing good or bad medical news.

The first time I sat vigil in the large Cedars-Sinai waiting room, I was wearing a summer dress and freezing. But now, for Michael's first cystoscopy with Dr. Mee, I wore Hard Tail workout pants and a sweatshirt, not only to keep warm but also to be able to do my mall-airport-hospital power-walking-the-halls for exercise. No reason not to multitask my health, especially when, as the caregiver, I couldn't afford to get sick. It was all about staying the course, keeping the faith, and making sure Michael got the best care possible, including my staying totally healthy.

I didn't know what to expect that first time I waited for Dr. Mee to tell us whether or not the prognosis from Michael's urologist Dr. Paul was legitimate. Michael's doctor hadn't seemed very thorough, so I was not surprised when Dr. Mee came out into the waiting room and said, "You guys were right. It looks like he has CIS. We won't have a definitive answer until the pathology report comes back in a few days, but I'm seeing something besides the inflammation from the last cystoscopy. I didn't think it would be the case based on the doctor's report, but it looks like CIS. I'm glad we went in. Somehow you knew."

The interesting thing about a diagnosis is that the worst day is the first day. After that, it's just putting one foot in front of the other as you figure out what to do. Both Michael and I are the type of people who want to know everything—the good, the bad, and the ugly. Whatever it is, bring it on. Tell us everything so that we know what we are dealing with. Spare no detail, let us know the whole truth and nothing but. Then we can decide our course of action based on all the facts. You can't stay on top of a protocol unless you're open to hearing every opinion and willing to read every pathology report. I've always been from the school of "knowledge is power, and once you know, you can't choose *not* to know." Michael makes jokes now about not being that kind of person before we got together, but I don't think that's true. He seemed only too willing to hear everything, which is much harder for the patient, because, let's face it—it is his or her life that's at stake.

While we waited for the lab results confirming Dr. Mee's professional observation that Michael did indeed have CIS, the plan was for him to start the first of six full-dose BCG treatments within the week while his bladder would be most receptive to the treatment. The days following Michael's July 24 cystoscopy were filled with as much real life as possible, plenty of research and praying and driving Nicky and Joey to and from the Marlborough School for their summer program. Taking everything from art to tennis to comedy to dance, the boys would spend from nine until three there every day while I sat in front of a computer learning as much as a could about bladder cancer. Never one to look only at the first page of search results, I gravitated toward the more obscure health-oriented sites that didn't have the budget to advertise. By reading anything and everything and being able to cross-connect a lot of varied and often opposing information, certain patterns begin to emerge.

Nicky and Joey's final performances at Marlborough were on the afternoon of July 29. I was sitting in the audience of Nicky's dance show when my phone rang and I was asked to hold for Dr. Mee. With my heart pounding and the curtain about to rise, she came on the line and explained that she had tried to reach Michael, but he wasn't answering his cell. She knew she had permission to tell me that the lab results confirmed that Michael *did* have CIS and it was worse than we had originally thought. She said, "Please have Michael call me tomorrow," as the lights went out and the curtain rose. I felt sucker punched in the stomach as the blood rushed to my head and I burst into tears. Then the music started and eighteen little girls began their hip-hop dance, and through my tears, I began laughing with joy and pride as I watched my nine-year-old son—the only boy up there—take centerstage and do his Justin

Timberlake–best as the star performer. The girls were screaming like he was one of the Beatles, and I couldn't help but feel, once again, that everything would be all right. Life is yin and yang, the good and the bad; it goes on, and Michael will be part of it.

Michael

The standard protocol for BCG is to inject it using a catheter into the bladder once a week for six consecutive weeks. To put it bluntly, it feels like swallowing a razor blade, and then pissing it out—it hurts! And no general anesthetic! First I had to lie down on a table with clinic paper covering my private parts. The nurse then painted my penis with a local anesthetic (not a very effective one, I might add) and clamped it. Next the nurse pushed the catheter in; a catheter is a long, plastic tube that goes into the head of the penis, then tickles past the prostate (not as fun as it sounds), and finally arrives in the bladder. The nurse squeezed thirty milliliters of the BCG solution into my bladder. The patient, me in this case, must hold the solution in the bladder for two hours, lying in various positions like a rotisserie chicken while the BCG works its magic. After this ordeal I was allowed to finally get up and urinate, and believe me when I tell you that never has a piss felt so bad and yet felt so good! By this time the bladder is shriveled up by the acidic action of the BCG and irritated to the point that I felt sick. And best of all, I'd get flulike symptoms, which took several days to pass, as well as painful urination that went on for days.

After all of this, one week later, the process began again. After the six treatments, there follows a month of rest, and then a cystoscopy to assess the effectiveness of the treatment. The month-long wait is so that the inflammation caused by the BCG has passed to the point where the examining doctor can see the tissue and assess the state of the cancer.

Around this time, I began to frequent a website called the Bladder Cancer Webcafé, which was a truly great website now gone dormant. Even if the Internet were not good for anything else, supportive online communities would still make it worthwhile. Thousands of sufferers and caregivers were given a forum where they could ask questions, share experiences, and learn to deal with their disease. When I joined this community, I was already beginning my new life and, as I read the posts each night, I saw how people differed in their approach to disease. Many of the people were persuaded by their doctors and their personal inclinations to seek easy answers. They would want the doctor to cure them, which invariably meant to cut out the cancer. Doctors across the country, many as misinformed as my first urologist, were urging patients to have their bladders removed to get rid of the cancer. As if the bladder is just some disposable sack that holds urine. As if each vital organ in the body does not perform a multitude of functions that make it nearly irreplaceable. As if the body is not an organism, but rather a collection of parts that can be discarded and replaced on a whim. These doctors are as foolish as their patients; together they destroy not only the lives of the sick but of the loved ones left behind.

I read about patients on the website who would be diagnosed with stage 1A (the earliest form, nonmetastasized bladder cancer) rejecting any treatment and insisting on having the offending organ cut out. And the doctors were not only obliging but also encouraging them! After a while, it became clear that many doctors were motivated by greed and aided by their own stupidity. To my eye this is criminal, but I guess it is really just negligence. As determined by many recent studies, many cancer patients in the United States would be better off never being diagnosed. And if they are diagnosed with cancer, they might be better off doing nothing rather than going to a conventional doctor for treatment. It says a lot that the vast majority of doctors would not go in for the conventional cancer treatment if they were the patient; they know how futile it is to cut, burn, poison the body to remove some errant growth whose cause can itself be treated.

Many patients on the website found love and encouragement and the strength to confront their disease and the difficult choices needed to find a cure that worked for them. They found information on how to deal with the effects of BCG, how to transition to healthier foods while not alienating their families, about the use of vitamin supplements to strengthen the immune system. This community of caregivers augmented my knowledge and helped me join the cancer patient community and feel that I was not alone.

I had been undergoing regular examinations with my new internist, Dr. Khalsa, with whom I developed a strong relationship. Due to his deep study of my body and the effects of the toxins he detected, he suspected that there might be more going on in my body than just the bladder cancer. Dr. Khalsa was proactive, unlike my previous physicians. He thought it would be a good idea to check for other possible cancers, just in case. It was now routine for me to spend more than half of my time in the vicinity of Cedars-Sinai Hospital in Los Angeles. On the day of my scans I went deep inside the hospital's windowless radiology department to get an EBCT, which is a scan of the heart and surrounding tissue and a CT scan of the chest. I lay down on the big cot to be slid in and out of the whirring machine, with a voice booming, "Breathe in . . . Hold your breath . . . Breathe!" When this was finally over, I got up and put my shirt on. The technician told me that I would have the results in a few days and that my doctor would call me.

I walked out into the next room and was met by a doctor. He asked me, "How did it come out?" I told him that I did not know, that I was told I would get the results in a few days. He cheerily said that he could look up the scan right now. I told him my name and birth date and he pulled up the EBCT. "Hmm," he said, "this looks pretty good. No plaque in the heart; see how clean that looks?" I looked over his shoulder, feeling a bit nervous. But then he said, "Wait, what about this dark spot down here?" He circled the spot and scratched his chin. "What other scan did you say you got?" he asked. I told him I had also had a chest scan. He pulled that up, and there was the dark spot again, a spidery looking mass of darker materials in my lower right lung. He then turned off the computer and said, "Don't worry about this; wait until you hear from your doctor."

Needless to say, I was freaked out as I walked through the hospital and out to the parking lot. When I got to my car I realized that I had left my cell phone in the scan room. So I retraced my steps through the labyrinthine hospital all the way back to that office. When I walked into the room, the same doctor had my scan up on the computer and was speaking to the radiologist. I heard him say that someone needed to examine this scan right away. He then noticed me standing there and clicked off the screen. I got my phone and went to my car.

Imagine the loneliness of that ride home. As I thought about what had happened, I squirmed in my seat. I let out a scream as so many thoughts raced through my head! I knew so much more about cancer then than I had when I was first diagnosed just two months before, and my newfound knowledge really scared me. Did I have lung cancer? Was that a spot on my lung?! Did I have metasta-sized bladder cancer? Was this the beginning of the end? Looking outside at the other cars, I realized how alone I was. My personal fear and agony were insignificant to anyone else except for Marilu and my children. I could die, and it would not affect anyone except them. No one would even learn anything from my fate—what was there to learn? The pettiness of my disease embarrassed me. I did not want Marilu to discover that I was even sicker than she thought. A sudden death by accident seemed soothing and alluring, but now that I knew I had a fatal disease I would never get that sort of pain-less death. Instead I felt fated to deteriorate slowly but surely, to dis-appoint all those whom I loved. My heart sank. The tears welled up in my eyes. I was totally screwed in a way that I had never imagined.

I thought back on my childhood and realized that there was no one hundred years for me. No living three score and ten. No seeing my granddaughter grow up. No old age, no marrying my true love. The finality of the situation made me feel so sorry for myself that I wept inside. I knew I had lung cancer without going to a pulmonol-ogist. I knew that my smoking had caused me to have an untimely death. I had brought this on myself. I felt like all the things I had done the past months, all the changes that had occurred after get-ting with Marilu, were for naught. A second cancer, possibly metas-tasized bladder cancer in the lung, would condemn me to an early death. My ignorance of what was important had led me to throw away everything.

But the human spirit is strong. The survival mechanism contin-ues to beat even in the breast of a condemned man. The dreams I had, snatched from long restless nights, were not the dreams of a dead man. I got to sleep each night with my beautiful woman, and that helped, but God, that ride home was still cold and lonely! I needed to see Marilu so badly, to hold her close and try to imagine this was not happening.

The drive home and those first hours were bad, the worst of my disease, as it turned out. So many people helped me through these two cancers—Marilu, my children, my parents, my doctors. But none of their help would have mattered without a strong internal desire to live. And not just a fear of death, though I had plenty of that. Through all of the pain and stress of my life, I remained an upbeat person. And now, as I faced death, hope returned to me. I could not give up! I had to try to live. And as I grew more resolute, my self-pity melted away. I would not be a victim; I would not give into this awful fate. Thank God for the power of denial. It gave me strength to ignore the odds and fight for my life.

When I got home from that horrific drive I called Marilu and gave her the preliminary report. There was nothing I could do now but wait for the radiologist to send in his findings and have a follow-up meeting with Dr. Khalsa. Nothing to do but ruminate, fret, and pace the floor. I had been a smoker, so lung cancer was an easy diagnosis. And a terrifying one! Of all my precious vital organs I had been the most cavalier with my lungs. The incessant smoking in my late teens and twenties—what had I been thinking? I had felt guilty, but yet I continued to suck that smoke deep into my lungs long after I stopped enjoying it. What an addictive waste that habit is! I finally quit in 1986 while on a business trip to Venezuela. I was left for a day with nothing to do, and so I had found a local bar and drank the wonderful local brew called Polar. And I smoked as I spoke the local language with the fishermen and truckers of Puerto Cabello and stared at the friendly polar bears lounging on the ice etched into the bottle. That night I had gone back to my hotel room, and there I spit phlegm into a wastebasket all night long. That was it. The chronic bronchitis finally convinced this old seaman to give up the habit. Now, seventeen years later, I not only had bladder cancer but possibly lung cancer as well! So much to regret.

Marilu

We were now on the fast track to see if the BCG could potentially cure the cancer, or at least hold it at bay while we let the detox do its magic and figure out what else could be done. Staging the cancer between 2 and 3, we knew that time was of the essence, so it was important that Michael stay the course with his detox, diet, supplements, and emotional wellness—including lots of happy, loving sex, of course. The night of his diagnosis we clung to each other, saying, "At least we now know what we're up against, and thank God we didn't wait until September." Hearing that Michael had CIS was definitely the scariest moment in our life together thus far, but it was soon outdone by more intense news the very next day.

Michael was driving back to his home in Palos Verdes when he called to say that during the CT scan Khalsa had ordered for his heart, they found a suspicious spot on his lung. Just when we thought we knew where he was at with the CIS, this new development could mean the worst news of all. We were in shock. His voice even sounded different as he was telling me the story. "I'll be right there," I said, not caring that it was rush-hour traffic and would take me two hours. I jumped in the car and put on the instrumental song "Inspiration" by the Gipsy Kings and listened to it again and again, saying over and over to myself, "If it's cancer, please just be lung cancer. Please just be lung cancer. Please just be lung cancer."

As crazy as that sounds now, I knew that if this new possible site were bladder cancer, it would mean that it had metastasized and would be even worse than our worst fears up until that point. And as if the music and mantra could ward off the cancer gods, I did not stop listening or repeating those words until I reached Michael's house.

For the first time since this whole ordeal began, Michael looked scared. We held each other close and couldn't let go. Neither of us said anything until, trying not to cry, I said, "Don't worry. Whatever it is, we will deal with it. Even if it's stage 4 bladder cancer, I've known people who have cured stage 4 cancers before. We will go all over the country to every place I know. You are not going to die."

Dealing with cancer is like a twelve-step program. One day at a time. Yesterday was the confirmation of CIS. Today was a spot on his lung. And tomorrow would be Michael's first BCG treatment. Who knew what that would bring? And all before we were leaving the day after that for San Mateo for another big BrownTrout party at his brother and sister-in-law's house. Michael's siblings and parents would all be there, and I wondered just how much he'd tell them about what he was going through. Michael comes off as the strong, silent type, but I knew none of this was going to be easy for him. *Listens to and follows directions*. With the spot on his lung, we'd now need more people to listen to and more directions to follow. But who were they? And what would they say?

CHAPTER NINE

August 1–26, 2003

Marilu

After a whirlwind week where each day felt like a body slam, Michael and I were on a Southwest Airlines flight to Oakland for the BrownTrout party weekend in San Mateo. The flight may have been less than an hour, but it felt like forever since it was the first time we could catch our breath and review what had transpired over the last few days. To be certain, there was a plan now in place that made us feel like we were on the right track—at least until further notice.

Just yesterday I had accompanied Michael to his first BCG treatment, and it was definitely stranger than expected. Watching the male nurse cover Michael's privates with a paper cloth, poke a hole in the paper large enough to expose his genitals, swathe the entire area with Betadine solution, tourniquet his penis with something that looked like a hairclip, inject a large plastic-holder shot of Valium directly into the tip of his penis, insert a long tube all the way into him so that it could journey over his prostate until it hit his bladder, allowing the BCG to be loaded directly into the bladder, and then filling him with thirty milliliters of liquid tuberculosis—

was hardly five-month-anniversary material. But I wouldn't have had it any other way. I loved every minute of being able to share and help guide Michael's journey to health. I can't tell you how many people at various times said to me, "You guys have only been together a few months? Why not bail?" Or "You don't have to stick around, you know. Not many people would." Or "He's probably going to die. Aren't you worried about investing too much time?"

I am never a quitter. I'm a mother lioness when I'm trying to protect someone I love. And I already loved Michael beyond any love I'd ever known.

The first BCG treatment gave Michael flulike symptoms, but he didn't want to miss the big BrownTrout weekend. We arrived late at night at the bed-and-breakfast that was housing Michael's family for the weekend in San Mateo, and even though it was after ten-thirty and most people were asleep, I wanted Michael to walk with me through the neighborhood to burn off energy and ensure a better night's sleep. Besides, a cool walk through a beautiful neighborhood seemed like the perfect time for us to discuss the party line on Michael's cancer information—just how much he would say and to whom. Many of his close family members had heard the most recent news about the CIS and spot on his lung, but this was a gathering filled with employees, and Michael didn't want to send anyone into a panic about the future of the company, especially when most people would probably not agree with the ways Michael was trying to help his body heal with vitamins, supplements, skin brushing, rebounding, colonics, detox, and a vegan diet. And daily exercise like a two-mile walk at midnight, of course.

The next morning, Michael's family was in rare form, especially his dad. Bill Brown was a true character, with William Powell looks and a Walter Cronkite voice. As complicated as his relationship with

Michael could be, it was obvious they both deeply loved each other. Bill was the kind of guy who started every day with whiskey in his morning coffee cup and continued sipping brandy throughout the day. He never seemed drunk, only more and more charmingly sentimental as the day wore on. Michael's mother, LaRae, a true beauty with a feisty personality and strong opinions, is the kind of woman who could have crossed the plains in a covered wagon while giving birth. It's no surprise that by twenty-two years old, she had three boys under the age of two and raised them by herself while Bill was in the Air Force. You want her on your team. And despite her being a pack-a-day smoker since she was a teenager, I hoped that she would be an ally in Michael's health quest.

The bed-and-breakfast hosts had made breakfast food to accommodate our dietary requests, a good time to test the waters of family support. There were the usual questions and comments: *Why no meat? No dairy? What do you eat? I could never do that. That's not what my doctor recommends.* Because I've happily lived this way since 1979, I never mind people questioning or scoffing at the way I eat; I know what works for me. And now I knew it would work for Michael, too. Getting his family on board might take awhile, that was evident. But as long as Michael was committed to changing his normal, I didn't care what they thought about his new way of eating.

That entire weekend, though, I didn't get the impression that anyone was taking Michael's situation very seriously. It wasn't just the meat and dairy and alcohol being consumed; it was the amount of chain smoking by several family members—almost as if in defiance of his cancer diagnosis—that felt disturbing. Not that Michael cared, but I did. Fair or not, everything in his life at that time was being evaluated by me as, *Is this potentially helping or harming*

him? Were the people in Michael's family making any connections between
what they ate, drank, or smoked to their health? What normal is Michael
used to that might need to be changed? Like an anthropologist studying
a tribe, I took notes on everything in Michael's world.

Michael

Upon receipt of the scans, Dr. Khalsa immediately sent me to the
pulmonologist Dr. Andrew Wachtel, who studied the scans and did
some X-rays and breathing tests. He learned my medical history
and about my active bladder cancer from Dr. Khalsa. Over time,
Dr. Wachtel became more than just a lung specialist; he became
part of the team that helped me navigate the healthcare systems
at Cedars-Sinai and other medical groups. Wachtel was open to
alternative treatments while also being very hard-nosed about the
science of disease. What I learned from him was that my lung condition existed outside the scope of modern medicine to easily diagnose in 2003. The dark spot shown on the scans could very well
be cancer, but there were other possibilities not easily dismissed.
Dr. Wachtel suggested we do "watchful waiting" and perhaps it
would go away. Who could refuse such an offer? Besides, with my
bladder just now undergoing treatment, who would want to open
another front in the cancer war? But it was hard. Now I had to visualize two hot spots, potentially two cancers, two areas of concern.
And I had to deal with regret, an emotion that tempts to inaction.

In addition to the BCG treatments, my new life also consisted
of constant detox treatments and regimens, some of which sound
exotic to me even now. I was full of toxins in my bladder, my liver,
and my skin, so I had to do something to clean these foreign com-

pounds out. Hydration was the single most important thing that I was missing. Taught by my father who bragged that he never drank water, I had never been much of a water drinker. I had given up sodas and such many years before but was just not accustomed to drinking much water. Now my diet was moving toward more, as Marilu calls them, *wet* foods like fruits, vegetables, and legumes that hydrate the body instead of sucking it dry. I added to my diet one ounce of water for every two ounces of body weight, or about one hundred ounces per day—the equivalent of about three-quarters of a gallon of mineral water.

My newfound hydration made possible the cleansing of my colon. Marilu had recommended I start colon therapy, and Dr. Khalsa referred me to a colon therapist named Laura in Venice, California. The clinic where Laura worked was simple, the room comfortable and clean. Laura was an African American born in the mining town of Douglas, Arizona. Her father had owned a restaurant in Douglas and later one in Silver City, New Mexico, both mining towns with large amounts of metal tailings in the groundwater. The toxins of mercury, arsenic, and lead found their way into the young children raised in these towns. From this hazardous beginning, Laura had then worked as an operating room nurse for more than forty years in hospitals, exposing herself to long hours, toxic chemicals, and unhealthy environments. She must have seen so much misery and death. Finally, she quit and turned to holistic health because of her own health issues, and eventually became a colon therapist after her own cleansing proved so therapeutic.

One of the beautiful things about embarking on a health journey is that people you would never meet otherwise become your friends, confidants, and mentors as you grope your way to a new and healthful future. Dear Laura became a friend, a guide, and an example. She changed her normal too late, as her body was consumed by a cancer that killed her very quickly, just a few years after we met. It is not always possible to undo decades of pollution and toxic stress. The body can heal itself, but it must be given time to reverse the effects of an unhealthy lifestyle. If I could help someone like Laura helped me, then that would be reason enough to write this book.

Laura gave me my first colon cleansing in July before I began the BCG treatments. Marilu had shared with me her positive experiences with colon therapy from the first time she tried it in 1981. The first time I went to the clinic, I was not that used to getting massages and the like, and colon therapy, also called colon hydration or cleansing, sounds a bit far out to most people. But Laura was so kind and professional; I looked forward to seeing her. At first I got a colonic every other day. Then, in the third week of going to see Laura, I had what she called a breakthrough. The colon treatment began normally enough, but once I was hooked up to the machine, I felt a rumble in my gut and then just started discharging. It was a sight to see. Up through the discharge tube went a lifetime of impacted fecal matter. This huge movement continued for the entire hour. I was not just having a bowel movement, I was letting everything go—all my repressed thoughts and feelings along with my fear, anger, and regret. As the eruption continued, the fecal matter kept coming out and going up the tube—seemingly everything buried in my past, encased in my gut, hidden from view came out—pizza from twenty years ago, old license plates, lost socks, even Jimmy Hoffa! I had a feeling of total physical relief. It was also the greatest sh*t of my life! At the end of my hour, I carefully got unhooked and went gingerly to the changing room. There I sat on the toilet for ten minutes letting go before getting up and dressing and hitting the restroom in the hall on my way out of the clinic. On the way home, I had to stop at a Del Taco and was in the restroom until they pounded on the door. I walked into the clinic that day with a size 42 belt, and after three days of releasing, I was a size 38. I had always suffered constipation, but no more. Laura finally flushed out the backed-up sewer of my gut and truly cleansed my polluted body. I feel like this was the moment that I truly began to heal.

Driven by my new career as a cancer patient, I launched a new life. Virtually every day I was getting tested or treated, either by a urologist, pulmonologist, oncologist, dermatologist, radiologist— you name it. And then there were the alternative treatments: the acupuncturist, the colon therapist, the lymphatic masseuse. The weeks were broken up by the Thursday BCG treatment, which laid me up for two days with flulike symptoms and a dilapidated urinary system. I felt like I was pouring Clorox through my bladder, down my urethra, and out into the toilet bowl. But by Saturday I was back to life and chasing Marilu for some intimate time. But with the BCG I was still toxic and had to be very careful, as the tuberculosis infection from the BCG could be contagious.

Every thought I had revolved around the fact that I had cancer. The name conjures up so many images, from the constellation in the night sky to the claws of the crab, to the aberrant cells growing unwanted and unchecked. To say I feared cancer was not accurate; I feared specific cancers. Had I drawn the long straw? Had my body done a good job in picking the lesser of so many greater evils? I did not know. I *did* know that bladder cancer is a bad one—maybe not as bad as pancreatic cancer, but neither was it as "good" as superficial melanoma. Visualization helped me to *see* all of this more clearly. The way the cancer spread in my bladder reminded me of corroded discharge pipes in an industrial chemical leach pond. The ends of the pipes corroded by the nasty acidic chemicals dripping out, the once round, smooth pipe now jagged and corrupted. My cancer had begun in the bladder proper, with the stalks growing like corn, and then later the CIS grew like moss on a tree down my urethra toward my penis. The toxic brew that had started the process must have sat on the delicate tissue of my bladder for far too long. From this toxic soup the errant cells sprang from healthy ones, and then had their own survival instinct that had to play out. My bladder was alive with a disfigured mass of tissue stuck like barnacles on the side of a ship. As those years of unchecked growth went by, the tumors that grew like stalks would leak blood from around their roots, which was the blood I saw in my urine those two years.

I had succeeded in visualizing this, of seeing into myself. Through months of visualization, of recurring thoughts about my urinary tract, I finally saw the ugly truth that was inside me. As I learned to see more clearly, my self-pity gave way to a renewed sense of love for this fragile vessel that I call my body. For so long I had taken it for granted and now, when it might be too late, I reached a place of love and appreciation. Is it inevitable that one comes to these realizations when it is too late? Thankfully, the only reason it was not too late for me was the love of one courageous woman, as well as her sense of health and balance.

In late August I was undergoing BCG treatments and had completed four of six weekly injections. During one of my weekly breaks I went with Marilu to Chicago and met with a doctor she has worked with since 1985, Dr. Keith Block, an integrative cancer specialist. Dr. Block advocates many of the same strategies as Dr. Khalsa but has an emphasis on food, and some other ideas that are his own. I went to him for a second opinion and felt better that he supported what I was doing in terms of detox and the use of BCG. I did not get into a discussion about my lung, as the bladder cancer was the focus at that time. Dr. Block gave me a renewed appreciation for the power of food and the need to change from a diet rich in sugar, such as fruit, to dark green leafy vegetables. I also saw in Dr. Block a kindred spirit, an adventurer with whom I could relate. He was an extreme surfer who surfed the Great Lakes in midwinter along with his hardy mates. Though the frigid lakes had never appealed to me as a seaman, I could definitely appreciate the adventure in surfing pounding waves of freshwater, the spray turning to ice as it is whipped by the wind.

Marilu and I were finally back in the city where we had first met. We stayed on the Northside in a loft owned by her sister JoAnn and her husband, Bill Drake. It was nice to be in Chicago with Marilu, and I was excited to go back down to Hyde Park where we had lived while going to the University of Chicago. Hyde Park back then had seemed dark and dangerous, except for the actual campus, but in the thirty years since, it had been totally transformed. We drove around our old college neighborhood feeling nostalgic because it felt like home. On the campus we visited the majestic Harper Library, but the most touching moment we had was when we went to the little Bond Chapel set just beside the *C* bench. I had loved this chapel when I was a student; it was a place I could go and enjoy the quiet. With the light streaming through the stained glass and the dark wood of the pews and altar, it was a soothing place. On our visit I realized that Marilu loved this place, too, and we even dared to talk about having our wedding there. But I was still being treated for bladder cancer and did not know about my lung, so planning a wedding seemed like a daring, even foolhardy, thing to do.

During this trip we continued to wait out the lung issue while healing (battling? fighting?) the bladder cancer. These terms always feel so off-target when talking about cancer and the love and care you must give your body. Unlike the cancer warriors you see on TV, I was not battling my body or trying to kill anything! I was trying to heal myself and find balance. I was visualizing that toxic waste dump in my bladder and trying to drain it, neutralize it, and make it a place where healthy tissues could grow. I loved my body, every part of it, yes, even the tumors that might kill me. Those tumors were a manifestation of my own imbalance, my own intemperate living. The BCG was forcing my immune system to rally in defense of my healthy cells, to steer the ship back onto a healthy course. All I had to do was supply the friendly currents, the warm breeze, and the calm waters of a stress-free environment to aid in my recovery. That was where my focus needed to be.

At Dr. Block's clinic in Chicago, people would come in for their chemo treatments and simultaneously get vitamin B drips and acupuncture and other alternative therapies. Their life force was nurtured and sustained while their body went through the trauma of chemotherapy. And why not? It seems so clear that we need to nourish the sick, not feed them ice cream sundaes. The medical community demonstrates its lack of understanding of food and nutrition in the simple act of accepting the quality of hospital food. What does this lack of care teach the patients? Are they supposed to take their diet seriously if the doctors and the hospitals do not? At almost every clinic in America where chemotherapy is administered, the only advice given on a regular basis for nutrition is *eat lots of protein*, meaning meat and dairy. What I saw at Dr. Block's clinic was another possibility, one in which people could be treated with these complex toxic chemicals at the same time as their body is being given a fighting chance by being nourished throughout the ordeal. I thought of my aunt, diagnosed with cervical cancer shortly after I was diagnosed with bladder cancer, who died just a few years later, her body totally ravaged by the cancer and by the chemotherapy itself. Her doctor couldn't wait for her to get back to normal, even if it killed her!

WHILE I FINISHED THE ROUND of six BCG treatments, I stayed at Marilu's house most of the time. This gave me the chance to get to know Nicky and Joey, and we gradually grew closer. Nick, nine at the time, was a very thoughtful, open young man. When talking to him you thought you were talking to an adult. He was very friendly with me, and he knew instinctively what subjects would interest me and would engage me in conversation. Joey, who was seven and a half, was smart and competitive and hooked on sports. He was very sweet, and I saw later that he, too, was a deep thinker. Both were brilliant boys who knew how to get along with each other without competing. I had had lots of experience with children and had suffered the defeat of many of my dreams for my own children. I think this made me more realistic than the average parent or stepparent, more forgiving, less demanding. I pledged to Marilu that I would never raise my voice at the children, and though I sometimes failed at this, I did find a way to be both supportive and accepting. As a result we bonded quickly so that by the summer, just months after Marilu and I got together, we were all one big happy family.

Watching life go on while feeling so vulnerable can be an unnerving experience. Certainly it can feel lonely, as it had on that ride home from the scan of my lungs. But it also can foster hope to rejoin the human race, to leave the cancer ward, if you can just visualize life on the other side. Hope is a good thing; it motivates us to go forward when otherwise we would give up. And so this new life with Marilu, this new family, nurtured me and gave me hope that I would have a life after the cancer.

Marilu

August became a series of weekly BCG treatments, Michael's visits to Dr. Khalsa, and getting my boys ready for their next school year. Booking Michael's BCG on Thursday meant that he stayed at our house for most of the weekend while he recovered, which gave the boys, Michael, and me an incredible opportunity to solidify our bond. There's nothing like a health crisis and a wicked game of Monopoly to really test the mettle of the man and how well he gets along with future stepchildren.

Michael's Thursday BCG treatments were getting progressively more debilitating as the weeks wore on, but as much as he took to his bed for forty-eight hours, he and I were ready for action by Saturday night. After a few rounds of BCG, Dr. Khalsa scolded us for having unprotected sex so soon after a treatment, but being baby boomers who became sexually active in the pre-AIDS sweet spot between the start of birth control pills and the era of *No Glove, No Love*, neither Michael nor I was even thinking about the dangers of the potentially toxic liquid tuberculosis and its effect on me. All we were thinking about was how much we wanted each other. Rightfully admonished, we decided to make it an adventure and try every type of fun condom we could find. The more that was thrown at us, the more we became a team that was up for anything. I never seriously, no matter what any doctor said or implied, or whatever horror story anyone told me or I read myself, thought for one second that Michael would not make it. Not. One. Second. I don't know whether or not I was kidding myself, or because of my memory I think I can see the future as well as the past, but I always had a vision in my mind of our being together many years.

Home-cooked healthy vegan meals, brisk walks around the neighborhood, lots of hydration, and by this time, I had gotten Michael into rebounding. Rebounding is basically low-impact movement on a minitrampoline. You barely have to move, and there is a handle to help you keep your balance, so anyone can do it. If you think of your body as highways of fluid that need to be circulated, rebounding is one of the best ways to stimulate your lymphatic system, or as I call it, *shake up the orange juice.* The most amazing thing about rebounding is that just two minutes of low-impact up-and-down movement triples your white blood cell count for the next hour. It also increases not only the oxygen levels throughout the body to even the most remote cells, but in addition, it increases lymph flow; improves cardio and respiratory function; fortifies bones; builds muscle; increases flexibility, coordination, and balance; and puts relatively little stress on the joints, soft tissue, and spine. It is one of the easiest, yet significant exercises you can do to improve your health.

After Michael's pulmonary doctor recommended a watchful waiting stance for the spot on his lung, I wanted to get a second opinion from another doctor I trusted. The boys were spending a week with Rob in Hawaii, so between Michael's fourth and fifth BCG treatments it was time to take the show on the road for a less than two-day trip to Chicago so he could be checked out by Dr. Keith Block, as well as meet two very special family members— my sister JoAnn and her husband, Drake—in the process. Returning to our University of Chicago roots was also on the agenda, and we couldn't wait to get on campus and compare notes about the various places that meant something to each of us. Strong memories are something I live with every day of my life, but to be with Michael, who lived and walked the same paths during the same time, so much so that I could literally take him to a spot and share a specific day and time and help him remember what he was doing at the exact same time was something I never thought I would get to do with someone, much less him. Beyond being surreal, it was profound. I felt like Emily in *Our Town*, only I didn't have to die to experience the reliving of the moment. We found our old classrooms and study spots and favorite hangouts and, when we got to Bond Chapel, we both looked at each other and simultaneously nodded in agreement, *This could be the place to get married!* Michael was being cautious, but I knew we'd be married one day, so whether it was Bond Chapel or Hacienda de Cortez in Cuernavaca, I was not afraid to talk about our future. Because I knew without a doubt we'd have one!

As much as we wanted to visit our old haunts on campus, I knew that, when it came time to eat dinner, it was more important to turn Michael on to my favorite vegan restaurant in town since 1983, the Chicago Diner, than to eat the food near campus that helped me stay overweight while a student. Sitting across from Michael in a booth I had sat in for thirty years, I marveled at the way he ordered now. He was truly learning to love the food that loved him and felt confident doing so. Every day we spent together I loved him more and more, and now, here we were in my hometown, in the city of our alma mater, and sharing a life we had lived so many lives to get to. That night we stayed at my sister and her husband's apartment above their photography studio. They weren't due back until the next evening when we'd all be having dinner together, so it was our perfect opportunity to role play campus lovers worried about getting caught. We couldn't believe we were in Chicago where it all began for us so many years ago. Sharing the city gave us a time continuum that not only connected us but also calmed our nerves.

The next day, Monday, August 25, I was excited to drive up beautiful Lake Shore Drive on our way to Evanston to meet Dr. Keith Block at his office, which is now called the Block Center for Integrative Cancer Treatment. Having known Dr. Block for twenty-eight years at that point, I trusted his cutting-edge ability to help people, especially cancer patients. Known as the father of integrative oncology, and long before almost any other doctor in the country, Dr. Block was famous for giving people vitamin drips to strengthen their immune systems before putting them through any kind of chemo, thereby keeping their health and, usually, their hair intact. Since 1985, Dr. Block was also responsible for the type of food his patients would receive at Presence St. Francis Hospital, making sure cancer and heart patients got miso soup instead of Jell-O, or brown rice instead of pork chops or Salisbury steak. Dr. Block was a handsome extreme sports enthusiast with tons of energy and married for many years to his fabulous wife, Penny, who was also a chef. Both Keith and Penny had been guests on *The Marilu Show* in 1994, and I had stayed in touch with them over the years.

I first met Dr. Block on Saturday, August 3, 1985, when I broke out in hives the night before and had no idea where they came from. I was still covered in hives the next morning and called a friend who knew about macrobiotics and the vegan lifestyle who said I should go see Dr. Block. He agreed to meet me in his office and instantly became a doctor whom I've stayed in touch with since. The day we met, I also met Dr. Robert Mendelsohn, who is the first doctor who talked about spacing out vaccinations so that the child is stronger when receiving them. For example, giving the three-month vaccinations at six months, the six-month vaccinations at a year, and so on. More than thirty years ago, Robert Mendelssohn made this recommendation, and I followed this protocol and never had a problem with my boys in terms of reactions to vaccinations.

Michael and Dr. Block hit it off. Kindred spirits. Long before it was fashionable, Keith's entire practice has always been the embodiment of integrative medicine, which looks at the total picture of the patient's life, or as his center currently describes it, "The treatment efficacy of conventional medicines can be enhanced when used in combination with supportive therapies such as a personalized nutrition plan, nutritional pharmacology, botanical medicine, psychosocial support, and improved physical conditioning." I was honored that day to find out that my first health book, *Total Health Makeover*, is one of the books they recommend to their patients.

We left the Block Center armed with additional supplements and Michael's greater appreciation for all I'd been telling him. (There's nothing like being validated by a credible institution!) Full of renewed hope, we headed out to dinner with my sister JoAnn and her husband, Bill Drake, and when Michael met Billy, a true bromance took root that, to this day, is one of the closest relationships among our extended family members. We headed back to LA the next morning in time for Michael's one-fifteen p.m. appointment with Dr. Khalsa, more determined to stay the course, and more in love than ever.

CHAPTER TEN

September 2003

Michael

W hile I was cleansing my body, I was having my weekly BCG treatments against the backdrop of a fuzzy diagnosis of possible lung cancer. Each week I would go through the routine of having the catheter inserted in my penis, the squirting of the thirty milliliters of solution, the two-hour wait, and then the pain, the nausea, the flulike symptoms, repeated again and again for six weeks. Finally after six weeks the treatments were over. I retreated into this netherworld where I was not doing treatments but still in therapy. I had no idea if the BCG had done anything. The fact is that some patients do not respond to immunotherapies such as BCG, and you never really know until you have tried them. Like so much of modern medicine this treatment does have a kind of hit-or-miss quality to it.

Even though I didn't know yet if the treatments had been effective, I was sure glad to be done with them for a while. The toll on the body is different for each person, and I must have tolerated it pretty well to do so many treatments. But since that day in July when Dr. "This Is Your Lucky Day" tried to sell me on bladder removal, there was no choice in my mind but to take the BCG treatments and try to save my organs.

I had a heightened sense of urgency in the way I was now detoxing my body on a daily basis. I was doing so many different things throughout the day: First there was the water I drank throughout the day, usually simple mineral water but sometimes mixed with green superfood. The bouncing on the rebounder, the skin brushing, the weekly colonic sessions. The daily infrared sauna worked to sweat out toxins from the skin and also helped with sleep. The iscador, which I injected every other day. And the nights were so effective, devoted to love of a special kind, where loving the night away in my lover's arms became my home and my escape.

But finally the interim period—between the sixth BCG treatment and a follow-up cystoscopy—was over. Again Marilu and I went to the hospital in the morning and checked in, and again they put me under with a full anesthetic. I woke thinking (hoping!) that Dr. Mee would tell me that I was cured, that it was a miracle, that no one had ever reacted this well to BCG and healed so quickly from bladder cancer!

But no, when Dr. Mee came in and told us the results, they were very discouraging. Basically, there had been no effect. She said that the bladder cancer might have advanced to the point where it was resisting the treatment. She told us that I could do another round of six treatments of BCG, but that the medical literature indicated that I should have the bladder removed at this point. There was always the chance with an active cancer that it would metastasize outside the bladder, making a recovery that much less likely. And besides, I now had this undiagnosed condition in my lung. There would be no easy decisions.

I had to decide whether to try another round of BCG or go

for the surgery. Decisions of this magnitude are best left to the patient. Even Dr. Khalsa could not tell me what to do, whether to follow the advice of the standard medical protocol and have my bladder and prostate removed, or to try another round of BCG treatments. I think that Dr. Khalsa knew that I was a very diligent patient and that I was pursuing the detox and immune system strengthening regime that he had laid out. But the responsibility for my health had to lie with me; it is my body, after all! And I just did not see life with a bag strapped to my side full of urine or a neobladder and inflatable balloon for a prostate as something I would choose under any circumstance. This reluctance to go there, to not consider major surgery, stemmed from my belief that once the surgery began it became a slippery slope toward a total physical breakdown. Each organ performs a multitude of functions, many of which modern medicine still does not understand, therefore I just did not see the value in surgery as a way to cure myself.

Marilu was by my side, and she told me we would make it work whichever way I decided to go. That was a great comfort to me. She was not pushing me to take the conventional wisdom or to make easy choices. But she was also not abandoning me to some crank treatments and quack doctors. She was supporting me in the best way possible, with information, honesty, and love.

Thank God I did not have my bladder and prostate removed but, instead, embarked on the second round of BCG, knowing it might be my last chance to avoid horrendous surgery. By this time, the lifestyle changes I had started began to have a noticeable effect. Each weekly treatment led me closer to the day when I would be scoped, when I'd see the outcome of all I had done to save myself. Visualization convinced me that I was on the right track; I was much more in tune with my body and more aware of the urinary tract and its components. I would visualize the urine secreting through my kidneys, draining into my bladder via the ureter, and then resting in my bladder before discharge. I knew the ways of my bladder, how it reacted to the BCG, and how it responded to days of rest. The copious amount of water constantly drained my bladder—my body was cleansing from the inside, and it made everything I was doing that much more effective.

It was great to have a routine to practice that could help my body get through this ordeal. The daily routine kept me calm and focused, allowed me to participate in my cure, to be responsible for my health. I was not a passive patient waiting for the doctor to figure out what to do with me. I was in charge of my treatment, with doctors as my caregivers.

In just four months, I had changed so much in the way that I related to my body. I had gone from the guy who let a lousy urologist lull me into complacency for two years to one who took control of my life and my medical treatment. Not because I was so smart or knowledgeable, but because I was the only one who could change my normal, and it had to be done thoroughly and quickly. I was the only one who could make myself skin brush in strange hotel rooms, search for vegan options in an Olive Garden, look for a colon therapist in Oregon.

I saw clearly what had caused my bladder cancer, and this made me confident that I could bring about positive change. I had decided to love my body more than my cancer did. This was not a war on some foreign entity; it was a family squabble that needed to be resolved. Once the anger left my body, and the BCG pointed the way for the immune system to do its job, the cancer was doomed.

After the second round of six weekly treatments of BCG, I waited again for a couple of weeks for what was to be my third cystoscopy in five months. Marilu and I both knew that a report indicating continued bladder cancer would probably mean drastic, life-changing surgery. But by this time our love was so strong, our commitment so complete, that I don't think either of us had any doubt about the outcome. Starting with the breakthrough with my colon cleansing in late July, my health had steadily improved. The confidence I felt from the detox and cleansing made me sure I was on the right track. As I went under one more time for the cystoscopy, I assured Marilu (and myself) that we would get a good report. When Dr. Mee and Marilu came to my bedside after the procedure, I could tell that the treatment had worked. And I knew that by changing my normal I had helped it to succeed.

The time from my diagnosis on May 22 to my *all clear* report on October 23 was a scant five months. The cancer had been growing in my bladder for years, but it was put into remission in a matter of months. I now was free to focus my full attention on the spot on my lung and to do so with more confidence than ever.

October 2003

Now that I had my all clear from the bladder cancer, my entire focus became the persistent dark spot on my lung first identified in late July. My pulmonologist was not sure it was cancer, as there were other possibilities, including a condition known as BOOP, bronchiolitis obliterans organizing pneumonia. So I had spent a couple of months watchfully waiting as I dealt with the bladder cancer. I was totally fine with watchful waiting; it made a lot of sense to me. I did not believe in a lot of the hocus-pocus that has been built up around cancer, believing instead that there is a logic to its growth and that much can be learned about a particular person's cancer by watching it over time. As I had now made my body much less hospitable to growing tumors, I felt even more comfortable watching and waiting, but some of my doctors thought I should get this mystery resolved now.

The usual way to diagnose a cancer is to take a sample and test it for malignancy. This was relatively simple for my bladder cancer, once I found a doctor who was thorough and engaged. But it wasn't so easy for the lung. The only way to get a sample of this lung mass without performing surgery was via a needle biopsy, in which the doctor inserts a long needle into the lung and sucks out a small piece of the dark mass. But it was very hard to reach the mass, and any negative biopsy result may only mean that the needle missed the target. Chest X-rays and MRIs were also ineffective, as they could identify the mass but not diagnose the condition.

One day on the phone I discussed with Dr. Block the difficulties of diagnosing my lung condition, and he suggested that he could perform a needle biopsy that would succeed. Marilu and I made a plan right away to go to Chicago to have the test done there.

My doctors in Los Angeles did not agree. This happens often when one gets a second opinion. I had thought, in my days of blessed ignorance, that there were standard procedures and proven therapies that all doctors agreed upon. Not so! Doctors seem to enjoy disagreeing with each other. Some can be very hard on their colleagues, questioning their skills, their wisdom, and even their motivations. This can be difficult for some patients, who may want to stop the madness and just go with their first doctor's advice so they can shut out the noise and conflicting opinions. It can also be hard on family and other caregivers, but is something that anyone facing serious surgery must go through if they want to maximize their chances of survival.

The patient who foregoes a second opinion is abdicating responsibility for their health to the doctor. The mind-set is, *If I just do what the doctor says, no one can say I didn't try, that I wasn't a good patient.* Due to this passivity, the patient may miss the chance to do the small things to change their normal that can make such big differences in the final outcomes of their disease. Without a second opinion, the patient misses out on the chance to get a different view of their disease and possible treatment. A specialist oftentimes will have a different opinion than a surgeon, who may have a different opinion than an internist. Dr. Khalsa served as my mediator, but I still had to make the ultimate decision myself, even if that decision was wrong. If a patient asks, *What else can I do, Doc?* the usual response is, *Nothing. The medical literature indicates this treatment if you want to have the best chance of survival. So just take your medications and get some rest, and try to eat. Don't worry about second opinions, we know what we are doing.* No discussion about diet, vitamins and supplements, detox strategies, or healing therapies, other than drug therapies. So sad; such a waste, to my mind!

By this time, in seeking all the answers I could, I'd met with a lung surgeon at Cedars-Sinai Hospital named Robert McKenna, who believed the best strategy was to put me under and do an arthroscopic procedure to remove a small part of my lung that included the mass and then biopsy it. McKenna was a renowned surgeon, and Dr. Khalsa felt like I should follow McKenna's advice. But I did not want to undergo any surgery that I might be able to avoid, and so—making the decision I thought was best for me—I followed Dr. Block's advice and went to Chicago to finally get a diagnosis of this lung thing without surgery.

October 27–November 15, 2003
Marilu

The spot sighted on Michael's lung was not yet clearly defined, and during the watchful-waiting period, we felt it was necessary for him to go once again to see Dr. Block in Chicago. We had the appointment set up for Tuesday, October 28, but, in the meantime, I was invited to the Louis Vuitton United Cancer Front Gala, which was, ironically, an event for cancer research. Lilly Tartikoff, who was married to the late Brandon Tartikoff, the former head of NBC and later Paramount, ran the prestigious gala. Lilly became a friend when my second husband, Rob Lieberman, and I ran into the Tartikoffs in Hawaii in September 1995, when Nick was a baby and I was seven months pregnant with Joey. I had already known and worked with Brandon during the final season of *Taxi*, and in 1988, I actually played a female character based on Brandon's early television career in the pilot *Channel 99*. He was a great guy, a true gentleman who loved the business and was taken away too young at forty-eight. After Brandon passed away from Hodgkin's lymphoma, Lilly became very much involved in cancer research. Along with Revlon CEO Ron Perlman, she founded the Fire and Ice Ball, which was always wall-to-wall celebrities and fabulous entertainment. The event in 2003 was as beautiful as always, and when I looked at my handsome date that night, I couldn't believe he was even remotely sick.

There was no way Michael and I could attend the event and be in

Chicago for Michael's needle biopsy the next day unless we flew the red-eye to Chicago. So there we were, leaving the ball long before the stroke of midnight. I was dressed in a beautiful light blue strapless Donna Karen gown and Michael in his fabulous black Armani tux that, by then, he'd gotten plenty of use out of, changing from the skin out while in the backseat of a limo tooling down the 405 to LAX. It's not easy going from a gown and tux to sweats and sneakers unless you've done it before, which I have, many times, in fact. Being an actor gives you practice with this type of thing; you learn to change your clothes quickly and discreetly, anywhere. Michael, however, had never been called upon to shield a half-naked female from the prying eyes of a limo driver. But we were on a mission to have it both ways—a fully realized Hollywood experience and a model patient on time and ready for surgery by nine a.m. Nothing ever stopped us from living our fullest lives. We were a team and somehow always managed to give 100 percent to every step of the process. Michael was the perfect patient. Not once, not even one time, did I ever hear him complain or express a *woe is me* attitude. He took every bit of information in stride and tried to make sense of what was happening with what each test, procedure, and doctor was telling him about his own body.

The red-eye brought us into Chicago around sixty-thirty a.m., and by seven-thirty we were ushered into a room where they would be prepping Michael for his nine a.m. surgery. At this point, we were already so comfortable being in hospitals that we had no compunction about asking, since we were about an hour early anyway, for a place to sleep for the extra hour or so. The nurse led us to an unoccupied hospital room, dark and windowless, but with a gurney large enough for the two of us to snuggle together and sleep a glorious extra hour and fifteen minutes. Not even the mixture of stiff, overstarched hospital bedding and antiseptic hospital smell could keep us from luxuriating in the moment. At this point, Michael and I were true partners in crime; madly in love and ready for anything. Each day was a matter of life and death, but we never thought we wouldn't have a happy ending.

The procedure du jour was a needle biopsy through Michael's back ribs and into the suspicious spot on his lower right lobe. Not an easy one to look forward to, but we wanted answers and this was one way of getting some.

So here we were, after our morning nap, with Michael getting prepped for a biopsy and Dr. Block feeling pretty confident that everything was going to be okay no matter the outcome of the procedure. After saying goodbye to both of them, I knew I had only a little time to hit the stores and buy something warmer than what we'd brought from LA as outerwear. Even though I'm a hometown girl, I'd forgotten how cold Chicago is by the end of October. I bought Michael a thick sweatshirt and a black pea jacket for myself that still hangs in my closet to this day, reminding me of those days in Chicago every time I look at it. I made it a point to buy something classic that would never go out of style. Just like us.

Michael's procedure was very short and ended early, as a matter of fact. When I went back to find him, he was already in the postoperative room, and Dr. Block came in to tell us the good news and the bad news. The good news was he still didn't know exactly what it was, but he couldn't say it was definitely cancer. And the bad news was that, because the lung is so delicate, the needle probe actually collapsed Michael's lung during the procedure. This risk is common, because the lung is like a balloon, and if you make a small hole in the balloon, air can escape from the hole and fill the space between the lung and the chest wall.

So there we were, stuck in Chicago with Michael unable to fly because of his collapsed lung, but I was in the middle of shooting the miniseries *Gone but Not Forgotten* in Sacramento with Brooke Shields, Scott Glenn, and Lou Diamond Phillips and had to be back on the set two days after Michael's operation. The clock was always ticking like a metronome in those days, giving a pace to our lives. This week was no exception. My boys were in school, I was due on the set, and Michael was stuck in Chicago with a collapsed lung. And to top it all off, it was Halloween week and, as any parent of schoolchildren knows, it's one of the most important weeks for projects and pageants. Originally the whole week had been worked out so that Michael could have his procedure on Tuesday, October 28, we'd fly back the twenty-ninth, I'd go back up to Sacramento to shoot on the thirtieth, be home for Halloween's school events and trick or treating, and then back to Sacramento on November 5 for more scenes.

But the key to your life is how well you deal with plan B.

And as we had told Dr. This Is Your Lucky Day, "We're a sexy couple!" So to make lemonade out of a lemon, we decided a train trip was the answer. Michael would hang out in Chicago recuperating while I flew back to the West Coast to shoot the miniseries in Sacramento and share Halloween with my boys in LA, and then I would fly back to Chicago so that Michael and I could take a three-day, two-night train trip on Amtrak's *Southwest Chief*. Very therapeutic and definitely romantic—the perfect solution.

Michael

Marilu and I arrived in Chicago on a cold morning in late October. We drove to Evanston and checked into St. Francis Hospital. There I was put on a bed facedown with instruments arrayed around me, including the long scope equipped with a needle poised above my back. They gave me morphine as I was going to be poked repeatedly, while also undergoing numerous X-rays to help position the needle and, hopefully, find the mysterious mass. They ran their tests, positioned the needle, and then poked me between the ribs and down into my lung. I could hear the whizzing of the mechanical arms as they moved above my head.

"Nope, missed it," one of the technicians said. Then they went in again and missed again.

And so it went until about the fifth time when someone said, "Oops, punctured his lung."

At that point I gasped out, "More morphine please!"

I was in the smooth twilight of a morphine drip and wondered with bemusement what a collapsed lung would feel like. Lying on my chest in the intense lighting of a movie set, with medical instruments and equipment around me, I struggled to notice that my right lung was flat like an empty balloon. As I breathed in I noticed a constriction as I inhaled, as if half my lungs were not working, which indeed they weren't. *If this is all it is then that's not too bad*, I thought, and I got to stay in the glow of the morphine awhile longer . . .

The needle biopsy had failed, but for reasons my doctors in LA had not anticipated. Would they have found the mass if they had continued? I will never know, as the procedure had to stop once I had a collapsed lung. I had tried one more time to avoid surgery, but it seemed that now I would have to go under the knife. I resigned myself to that fact as best I could.

Marilu had to rush back to Los Angeles the next day to be with the boys and shoot her miniseries, and I could not go with her because I could not fly for thirty days, the common precaution for those with collapsed lungs because of the possibility of cabin depressurization. So Marilu left, and I stayed in Evanston while waiting for her to return so that we could take the train home together from Chicago to Los Angeles. This was a strange time for me, as I was in quite a delicate condition and was left by myself with nothing really to do for three days. My body was still recovering from the BCG treatments, and I was deep into the process of dealing with the mass in my lung. I walked around Evanston and spent a lot of time in a cavernous bookstore in the center of town. I worked by phone and Internet. I went to the Bladder Cancer Webcafé to talk about my experience and discuss what to do next after getting an all clear from the urologist. I did not begrudge the doctor who had brought me to Chicago. I had wanted to avoid surgery, and he agreed to try to help me. The fact that it did not work was a risk I had been willing to take.

Marilu's sister JoAnn and her husband, Billy, happened to be in town. I visited with them and told them about our plans for a train trip to Los Angeles. Billy was pretty skeptical of the comforts of a cross-country train leaving from Union Station, but both Marilu and I looked forward to this time alone together. I see in Billy a man with a great attitude toward life, which makes him fun and attractive. He bounces around, dancing and laughing, always ready to be part of the party. This attitude of his, his love for life, seems to contribute to his amazing stamina, as he now is in his eighties and going strong. If only I'd had the balance and passion to live my life like Billy, I might never have gotten cancer!

I walked the streets of Chicago on Halloween night as I waited for Marilu to return from LA. I wanted to get out and see the city, so I went to the near Northside and then walked up Clark Street. The city was so different from when I had lived there in the seventies and drove a yellow cab. The world had gone from pre-*Taxi* to post-*Seinfeld*. I felt much more like a mortal than I had been then, all full of life and in a hurry. Back then I would go to the cab barn at Fifty-First Street and Cottage Grove, definitely a shaky neighborhood, and drive my cab up to the Loop. There I would hang out, picking up conventioneers and shuttling them between bars in Chicago and Cicero, where the barmen would pay five dollars a head for each guy I brought in. I was in a hustling mood in those days. Now I was reflective, letting memories wash over me as I walked up the frigid street, avoiding guys dressed like superheroes and women dressed as French maids.

I missed Marilu that night. Halloweens to come I would be with her and the boys, trick or treating around our friend's neighborhood. But this night I walked around alone and missed my baby. Even though I still did not know what was in my lung, at least now I knew what I would do to find out. I decided that I would go through with the surgery as Dr. McKenna had recommended and finally find out exactly what was going on in my lower right lung. It felt good to finally find my direction, to know what my next treatment was going to be. But this direction was one I had dreaded, because in my heart of hearts, I knew I had lung cancer. The only question for me was whether it was metastasized bladder cancer or a completely new cancer site. And then, whether or not the tumor could be removed surgically so that all of the errant cells were gone and there were only *clean margins*. If there were errant cells left over, there was the chance that they could later grow into another tumor or metastasize elsewhere in my body.

There was another reason that I had avoided the surgery for so long, why I dreaded it so: I was stubborn and just did not want to lose any piece of myself. By now, after more than five months of cancer and the hard choices I had already made, I would have felt defeated if I then lost part or all of my lung to cancer. I was fifty-one. I kept thinking that if I dug this organ out here, or cut that one off there, that eventually I would not be alive, or that my life would not be worth living. I had just barely beaten the bladder cancer; it had been only a week since my all clear cystoscopy. And now I had to go under the knife for real.

In addition to the lung spot there were the ongoing treatments to prevent recurrence of the bladder cancer. I had researched this and knew that I was going to have to submit to BCG treatments every three months, with cystoscopies after each treatment, for years and years. This was because I was going to follow the protocol of Dr. Donald Lamm, who had studied the long-term effectiveness of BCG for maintenance of patients who have had bladder cancer that's been put into remission. His protocol helped me to understand that cancer is indeed a chronic disease, that no patient is ever "cured." This did not scare me, because my changing normal was a lifelong undertaking, and this maintenance of my bladder was just part of that.

But now I had to consider what would be the result of a lung surgery where I would lose one of the lobes, or about one-fifth of my total lung capacity? Or even the entire right lung? How would that feel? How would it affect my long-term survival? What long-term maintenance would I need then? Couldn't I just cure this lung cancer through a healthy diet and clean, stress-free living?

I finished my walk through the Northside and retired to my hotel. I looked forward to Marilu arriving the next day and our heading west on our train trip. I would put all of these fears in the back of my head, out of sight, so I could enjoy the trip. After all, who knew how many more such trips Marilu and I would be able to take?

THE NEXT DAY MARILU AND I headed to Union Station. I had been there so many times as a student arriving from or going to Salt Lake City and as a cabdriver picking up fares and taking them out to the suburbs. It looked like it had in the seventies, gray and cavernous, just like what the main Chicago train station should feel and look like. We huddled on a bench and waited for our train. The porters were gracious and led us to our cabin. We had a couch that pulled out into a full bed—what's not to like? We ordered a bottle of wine and pulled out of the station. Heading west, we reached the prairie just as the sun set. Marilu and I held hands and looked out at the Great Plains. It felt like we were at the beginning of a long journey, like we were going to be together forever. That is what I thought, and I told her. I wanted to let her know that I was in for the long haul—that I would get through this with her love. But I held off on a proposal. I felt like I had to get clean from all of my cancers before I would feel right asking Marilu to marry me.

I lay in bed that night and slept like a seaman in his rack, but instead of the tide gently rolling, it was the steady clack of the wheels that put me to sleep. In the early godforsaken hours before dawn I woke up as I felt the train lunge to a stop. I raised the blind to see the backside of downtown Kansas City. Such a romantic stop, I could not help but wake Marilu to see it! In their heyday the great

train stations had the best of downtown facing them with giant bill-
boards luring the train travelers. Now it was dilapidated, but you
could still see the grandeur that had once been there.

We switched cars and engines in Kansas City and then moved
on across the Missouri River. As the sun rose, we went to breakfast
in Kansas. We lounged in our car and read our books. As we rolled
down south toward New Mexico and the evening came, we wanted
to light a candle. Our porter did not have any matches, so I went
to the smoking car to bum a light. Such a strange experience! The
smoking car had stainless steel walls and ceiling with bright lights.
The poor fools stuck in there smoking did not appear to be having
a good time. The smoke and the ashes and stainless steel made it
feel like a giant ashtray. I thought about how smoking had most
likely shortened my life; there was no denying it. And to think that
I had given up years of my precious life to this stinking, pointless
habit! I had to feel some big regret no matter how much I tried
to put those thoughts away. Heading back to our cabin with the
matches, I resolved not to waste what good times I had left with
regrets and doubts. It made me laugh to think how horrible the
smoking experience was on that train. Maybe if I had been rele-
gated to that smoking car back in 1970 I would have quit smoking
then and there!

I lit the candle and we turned off the light. The door was shut
and the car was quiet, except for the click-clack of the wheels be-
neath us. I held Marilu's hand in the dark and thought how lucky
I was to be alive and on this trip. A short time before, just eight
months, I was growing tumors and didn't even know it. And I'd
been alone without a woman to care for or to care for me. How fast
things had changed, and how completely! We made love on that
train that night, passionately yet quietly, beautiful. As I went to

sleep that night, I slept like I hadn't since I'd lain at anchor off the coast of Brazil.

The next morning we arrived in Albuquerque for our only time off the train the entire journey. We were in old downtown, not a great spot. Marilu had hoped we could get something different to eat, maybe something a bit healthier. But this was not the place to be looking for brown rice and vegetables. We got back on the train for the long pull up the mountains through Flagstaff and then down to LA. I felt closer to Marilu at that time than I had ever been with anyone. We had made this inconvenient train trip into something really special, and I knew her love was helping to cure me.

Marilu

Leaving Michael in Chicago the day after his collapsed lung drama wasn't easy, but I had to make it to Sacramento to shoot a scene where my character, a detective on the trail of a serial killer, breaks into a hotel room and finds the killer's stakeout. It was a late-evening shoot, but the ever-accommodating production team promised they'd do their best to wrap me in time to make the last flight out of Sacramento. That way I could be home in the morning to get my kids dressed and ready for their classrooms' Halloween festivities, because not only do I love all school activities, but as room mom for Nicky's fourth-grade class, I was responsible for making sure his Halloween Poetry Reading Event went off without a hitch. My boys are very different kids, as evidenced by their particular choice of costumes, that year especially: Nick went as Mozart, and Joey as a cop. And the Poetry Reading Event was a huge success!

The events during the few days away from Michael fell into place, but I was anxious to be with him again and start our trip back to LA to get answers. We knew something was growing in his lung; we just weren't sure what it was or what to do about it. As a research junkie I was hoping that if Michael did indeed have lung cancer, it was the non-small cell, slow-growing kind rather than the small cell faster-growing type of cancer, and that it was found early enough to be a stage 1 lung cancer rather than a stage 3 bladder cancer. No lung cancer is ever preferred, but in light of Michael's stage 2 to 3 bladder cancer diagnosis, the worst we could hear would be that the spot on his lung wasn't lung cancer at all, but rather metastasized bladder cancer.

But for now, we were just two lovers on a cross-country train enjoying a throwback experience, taking in the countryside and hanging onto each other for dear life. Each day is a gift when you're fighting the clock, and three days on a train gave us the opportunity to take stock, explore the possible outcomes, and plan our next moves. The one thing we could count on at that point was that we were in this together no matter what and so close that we didn't even need to pull down the second bed in our sleeper car.

Upon arriving at Union Station in Los Angeles, I was immediately picked up by a production vehicle and taken to LAX for another flight to Sacramento for more scenes of *Gone but Not Forgotten*. When you're shooting a miniseries and you're not the lead character, there is often a back and forth to your shooting schedule. I didn't mind making the eight trips to and from Sacramento because it afforded me the time to be with my kids and accompany Michael to his many appointments. But because it was post-9/11 and I was always booked on a one-way ticket, I had to withstand a full-body search each time. By trip number three, the Southwest

Airlines TSA gang knew my name and my Cosabella thong underwear, which always seemed to get caught during the waistband-checking part of the probe.

While Michael waited for his next appointment with his lung specialist, Dr. McKenna, my boys were able to spend time with their dad, who was in town for a short period of time, and I was in Sacramento for a few days shooting the most intense part of the miniseries. My character discovers a barn full of torture devices and three women who have been blindfolded, tied up, and brutalized by the killer. But it's always hard to be an actor in the middle of a fictional piece when what's happening in your real life is more compelling: At the very moment we were shooting the part when my character pulls up to the barn, I got a call from Michael. His daughter had been in a terrible physical fight with her husband, and she and her daughter, Michael's seven-year-old granddaughter, were now moving into his house. Within days, his other daughter also moved into Michael's home to get away from her boyfriend— not an ideal stress-relieving situation, but at least both girls were safe. With all the craziness between flying to and from the various miniseries locations and everything that was going on with our families and Michael's health, once again, show business paled in comparison to real life. I always say you can have it all if three things are in place: good people, good health, and good organization. Thank God for great kids, a strong constitution, and an organized carry-on.

CHAPTER ELEVEN

November 2003

Michael

I now began in earnest to get ready for the lung surgery, even though I did not know what to expect at all. The surgeries I had had so far were merely scopes and resections, not full-blown invasive surgeries. I did not know how much surgery could hurt, and you really cannot know until you've had one. I went to see Dr. McKenna, who examined me again. During our talk he told me that he thought I had cancer, and if it was lung cancer that he would get it out. I told him again that I did not want to lose any of my lung unless it was absolutely necessary, and he assured me that he would comply with my request. He was very confident and seemed to know how this would come out. He was not into alternative treatments and told Marilu that I could get back to eating whatever I wanted after my surgery. I was learning to take what I could from doctors and not look for more than they had to give. Surgeons are a strange breed, anyway: They do what others only talk or write about. They have a certain bravado that I guess they must have in order to take other people's lives into their hands confidently many times a week, fiddling with others' insides.

While waiting for my day of surgery I continued to work at the office, but to be honest I was more involved in my health journey than ever. I so wanted to be healed, but I thought that even the life I was then leading was not so bad. My physical health was improving, the bladder cancer was in remission, and I would soon solve the puzzle of the mass in my lung. I felt like I could survive the lung cancer, just like I had survived the bladder cancer. And maybe I would be even stronger as a result. But the doubts persisted because so many others doubted me. Two cancers at once, how did I know there was not another one lurking somewhere? I'd had skin lesions that were pre-cancerous. What about my lymph nodes? And then how did I know that I would not get a recurrence of the bladder cancer? How did I know what they would find when they started digging in my lungs? I tried to stay positive, to visualize a healthy outcome. But knowing how I had abused my poor lungs, so damaged by smoking and God knows what else, made me scared.

One good thing was that my family was very supportive. Despite the anger I had felt toward my father, he supported me, as did my concerned mother. My daughters were very sweet, and my son worried about his dad. It was very important to me that my family understood what I was going through and how much I loved them. I did not want my children to suffer, but I held out hope that they could learn from my experience, and I think they did.

At this time I also went to an allergist, who tested me with thirty-two pinpricks on my back. No allergies that he could find, but he still had me come back for one test after another. Finally I asked him what exactly he was looking for; he turned to me and said that he was trying to determine whether I had emphysema. My grandfather had died of emphysema. I looked it up. Emphysema is a condition of dead air linings in the lung tissue. God, did I regret the smoking!

I went through an extensive preoperative routine that included visits to my pulmonologist, Dr. Wachtel, and my internist, Dr. Khalsa. Everyone assured me what a great surgeon Dr. McKenna was, and I was quite confident in his ability. Still, I regretted the fact that I was going to lose some or all of my lung. I felt like I would never be whole again, and I so wanted to be whole, to have a chance to live a long life. But there was nothing to be done but submit to the surgery. I had exhausted every logical alternative.

Marilu drove me to the hospital that morning at five-thirty a.m. Always so early to check-in. The endless repetitive questions, the plastic strap around the wrist, the bogus fully clothed weigh-in, and the hurried blood pressure test. After saying goodbye to Marilu and entering the pre-op area, I was led to a bed and hooked up to the IV and monitoring machines. I lay there listening to the interns and nurses making jokes about Dr. McKenna. It seems that McKenna was a country music fan, and they had rigged up a speaker so they could play a tune for him. They were laughing and joking and ignoring me across the room. I played a trick on them just to have something to do, to show them that I was there with them. At that time, inexplicably, I had an extremely slow pulse. My average was in the midforties, and each time I got tested the nurse would ask me if I was an athlete or something. As I lay on that bed I could see the pulse monitor, and if I lay real still I could slow my pulse below forty-five, at which point the alarm would go off and the nurses would rush over. Something to pass the time. I guess if I could get my pulse down that far I must have been pretty mellow in that operating room!

Finally the anesthesiologist came in and prepared me for the anesthesia. I knew that once he shot me up the surgery I had dreaded for so long would happen. Trying to calm my fears as he gave me my injection, I faded out to the sound of twanging guitars and the interns welcoming the surgeon.

In case I did have cancer, I had arranged on Dr. Block's advice for part of my tumor to be rushed to a lab, where it would be subjected to several chemotherapies to determine the most effective one in case I had to follow up the surgery with chemo as a way to further ensure that the cancer did not spread. This was just another precaution, as I had only one chance to have my tumor examined before it was flushed down the toilet. I wish I could have seen it; it was part of me after all! But such curiosity seemed morbid to the hospital staff, and maybe it was.

From what I heard later, I know that the doctor went in through a couple of holes in my right underarm and, through a scope, found the mass and removed part of it. They hurried it to the lab, where a quick biopsy revealed cancer, bronchioloalveolar. Dr. McKenna went back in and removed the remainder of the lower lobe of my right lung and some lymph nodes. The margins were clean and there was a good chance that the cancer had not spread, that he had gotten all of it. The lymph nodes were biopsied and were shown to be clean of cancer cells.

I awoke in the recovery room groggy and in pain. I turned my head and saw Marilu sitting beside me. She told me that they had removed the tumor along with the lower lobe, and that they had gotten all of it. I was overcome with love and emotion. She looked so kind and gentle, so concerned, so loving. She had been through a lot with me in the short time we had been together. I grabbed her hand and thanked her for being there for me. We had talked about marriage almost from the time we had gotten together, but now it seemed we were through this horror show and heading for the exit. We had made it! And now I could commit, I could dare to love, and to think about the future. And so I rose up in my bed as best I could, strapped down as I was by tubes and wires, and asked Marilu to be my wife.

November 24, 2003
Marilu

Today's the day. Monday, November 24, 2003. Michael's lung surgery.

Neither of us slept well the night before, but even a few hours in each other's arms felt like eight hours anywhere else. We moved about the house quietly so as not to wake the boys or the babysitter who'd slept over to drive them to school. I'd be picking them up after school, because with Michael's six a.m. check-in and eight a.m. surgery, I was sure he'd be stable enough by three o'clock for me to take the boys shopping for what they needed for their school's Multicultural Feast the next day. It was Nicky's class that was putting it on, and he was representing Greece with an authentic costume we borrowed from the *Hellenic Times*, from whom I had received an honor in 1998 at their Hellenic Times Scholarship Fund Gala. Michael, the boys, and I had gotten into a family groove, and it was important to both Michael and me to keep our lives as normal as possible under the circumstances. Life is always action-packed during this time of year, but especially when you're trying to balance school, work, the holidays, and saving a life!

I had packed the necessary waiting room goodies—books, magazines, chargers, healthy snacks, and so on, paying extra attention to bring additional big scarves and sweaters for anyone who might be homesteading with me waiting for news from Michael's doctor. Cassia was set to be there as soon as she dropped Victoria off at school, and since it was her first time sitting vigil, I was sure she wouldn't bring warm enough clothes for a cold November waiting room stay.

It was still pitch-black when we arrived at the hospital, but we were old pros by now at getting up early and speeding up the process of checking in, especially once Michael had filled in all of his Advance Healthcare Directive paperwork designating me the person in charge. It's a big responsibility being the one who can make those life and death decisions, but neither of us would have had it any other way. I knew that Michael didn't want to lose any more of his lung than was absolutely necessary, and he was trusting me to make sure Dr. McKenna honored his request. When we saw McKenna that morning, we both reminded him ad nauseam about being careful. He gave us the look most people give me when I'm snoopervising their jobs, but I didn't care. I'm glad I'm pushy. And I had to say it out loud before Michael went under so that he knew I had his back. McKenna again reassured us that he'd do only what was necessary and went to scrub up. Michael and I kissed one last time before his anesthesia took effect, and there was no doubt in my mind that he would be okay. I could see our future in his face that still looked handsome, despite the ridiculous hospital shower cap they make surgery patients wear. I watched them wheel him away and said a little prayer before leaving the pre-op room to go pick my spot in the main waiting room.

By now many of the hospital staff and volunteers recognized us as regulars, and some even called us by name. One in particular was a huge *Taxi* fan and allowed me to keep my wheelie bag of supplies behind the desk while I power-walked the hospital corridors. I tried not to take advantage too often, but it was sure nice to be able to burn off some energy while Dr. McKenna did his magic. By the time Cassia arrived to sit vigil and wait for news with me, I felt revved up and emotionally ready to hear anything. The two of us watched the comings and goings of volunteers, medical personnel, and patients with hopeful anticipation, trying to read the expressions on each doctor's face when he or she came to deliver the sad or happy news.

When the door swung open and there was McKenna, Cassia and I jumped up and practically leaped into his arms. With his cowboy swagger and poker face delivery, it was hard to get a reading right away, but I did hear him say, "It went well. It was cancer, but it was in a convenient spot. I only took what I had to. The small lowest lobe of his right lung. Clean margins. I got it all." Cassia and I screamed, and through my tears I dared to ask, "Will I get ten more years with Michael?" McKenna scoffed, "Ten? I hope you like this guy 'cause you could get over thirty!" And when an uncharacteristically slight smile came to his face, I gave him a huge hug and lots of thank yous, no longer caring that I was invading his personal space.

He then went on to tell us that the cancer looked like stage 1A bronchioloalveolar lung cancer, not bladder cancer, and that he'd have the definitive results later this week, probably after the holiday. It was three days before Thanksgiving, after all, and I couldn't think of anything I could be more thankful for. It was not bladder cancer. It. Was. *Not*. Metastasized. Bladder. Cancer.

McKenna said his goodbyes and told Cassia and me that he'd check-in later that day and that Michael was in the first post-op recovery room and would be moved to the second one, where we could go back and see him in an hour or so. Cassia had to leave before then, so when she headed out, I went to my *Taxi* buddy volunteer and told him the good news. I wasn't *quite* trying to use the Force on him, but I wasn't surprised when he whispered, "Wanna go back and see him? Follow me."

I had been in the second post-op room many times after Michael's cystoscopies and other people's surgeries, but I had never visited the inner sanctum that looked almost like the scene in *Coma* with its still bodies, blue lighting, and complete silence, save for the beeps of the monitors. There were no other patients near Michael's bed, and he was still out cold, so I quietly tiptoed over and sat on the edge of his bed. Despite the oxygen tube in his nose, the bandages covering his obvious wound, and the various medical apparatus attached to his body, he still looked like a sleeping god. And seeing him in that state reminded me of my mother in the hospital, so many years ago, trying to survive the best we knew how at the time, and only wished I knew then what I know now. I could have inspired her with the same knowledge Michael discovered to save himself.

I sat there staring at his handsome face for about fifteen minutes, when he started to come to. His eyes blinked and then began to focus. I quietly said, "Hey, baby. It wasn't bladder cancer. It was stage 1A lung cancer. The good one. And McKenna got it all. He said I'll have you around for at least thirty years." He smiled and slowly slid his hand to mine, swallowed to clear his throat, and said:

"Will you marry me?"

Of course I said, "*Yes!*"

I couldn't wait to tell the boys the double-great news. Michael was going to be around for a long time *and* we were going to get married. Nicky was right—it wasn't a question of *if*; it was only a matter of *when*.

I brought the boys to the hospital to visit Michael on Tuesday after their school's Multicultural Feast was a huge success. And by Wednesday, barely fifty hours after his operation, Michael was going home. On Thanksgiving, he was still recuperating and could barely eat, but by Friday he woke up feeling stronger and more resolved than ever to live a healthy, long life. He was feeling so good, in fact, that that evening he was feeling frisky enough to have sex— four days after major surgery. What a guy!

Michael

Having trouble breathing and groggy from the drugs and the oncoming pain, I laid on the bed hooked up to monitors with a breathing tube hanging out my nose and a mass of gauze on my chest. The light in the room was nice, no windows, a warm glow. So when I looked at Marilu, and we both realized that we had come through this together it was natural to ask her to marry me. I croaked it out as best I could, and when she heard me she cried and touched me. She told me that my daughter Cassia had been out in the waiting room and would be so happy to hear the good news later on. The nurses then pushed my bed into my suite and hooked me up to the machines again.

I passed a few days in the hospital, and then it was time to be discharged. I was not sure I was ready, but the policy was to get the patients discharged quickly. Marilu took me home that afternoon and I took to my bed. The next day was Thanksgiving, and I managed to eat with the family. But that weekend I got a terrible cold. As I lay on the bed I felt the vacuum in my right lung, a hole in my chest. I closed my eyes and could visualize the empty space, with webs of blood vessels and nerve endings dangling in the void. The empty feeling persisted for a year as the middle lobe grew down and gradually filled in the space. But some lung capacity was lost forever and my famously low pulse rate changed to a more normal range in the sixties. No more messing with the nurses with that trick of mine!

I was so glad to be home, to be with Marilu and my family. All of our kids were happy to know that Marilu and I were engaged; it seemed like such a natural conclusion to such a dramatic journey. Normal for me had become a place of balance, a peace with myself and my body. Marilu told me that Dr. McKenna said that I could last thirty more years, and I was determined to give it a go. And with Marilu by my side I knew that I would get what I needed.

Marilu

Michael and I have been together for more than thirteen years now, married for more than nine, and his cancers have been in remission for more than twelve. Twelve years of glorious health. Every time he sees a doctor and gets another "all clear," I thank God and marvel at my husband's amazing ability to have changed his normal and saved his life.

Our wedding on Thursday, December 21, 2006, was a family affair: my sister Christal was my maid of honor; her nine-year-old musically gifted twins, William and Christopher, played cello and violin; Michael's brother Rob was his best man; his twin brother, Marc, officiated; my brother Lorin gave the wedding speech; Nick and Joey gave me away; and Jackson, born the day of Michael's and my first date, was the ring bearer. In addition to the standard wedding vows, I promised Michael that I would always pack for him, help take care of his dog Pablo, and love his children like they were my own. And Michael vowed he would agree to cohost our annual Henner Family Christmas, at least *try* to be on time, and to always follow the rules of the *Total Health Makeover.*

When I am asked to speak on various health topics at events all over the country, no matter what I am there to lecture about, after telling Michael's story, it's the only thing anyone wants to discuss. People are shocked and want to hear more. You can see from the look in their eyes that they have not heard most of this information before, but feel that, for maybe the first time, they are hearing some truths.

There is currently what I call the *tsunami of health.* Nothing can stop it. People are demanding answers. And thank God there are people like Dr. Neal Barnard from PCRM (Physicians Committee for Responsible Medicine), Nelson and Dr. T. Colin Campbell, authors of *The China Study*, and of course, Dr. Soram Khalsa leading the way. What I learned from so many wonderful sources in the seventies is becoming mainstream now, and I couldn't be happier.

And I couldn't be happier sharing my days with a beautiful extended family, two college boys who are not brats, and a healthy, happy relationship with the fearless love of my life.

CHAPTER TWELVE

2010-2011

Michael

W hen my father first heard about my bladder cancer diagnosis he sat down in his study and cried. How a parent must feel when their child is diagnosed with a deadly disease I do not know, but I can imagine. Because when my father was diagnosed with bladder cancer several years later I also wanted to cry. I wanted to cry for myself, for my father, for my mother, and for the whole world of tired actors moving through their roles and heading off the stage of life to meet their fates. My father did not have to die from bladder cancer, though die he did, and the reasons are far more complex than that he was diagnosed late and that he was in his eighties and that he refused some medical treatments and could not tolerate others. No, my father died prematurely from a cancer he could have avoided or mitigated, because he would not change his normal.

My father's cancer came at a time when he felt like he was my mother's caregiver. Because he felt so responsible for her he insisted that he must undergo radical surgery, give up his bladder and prostate, so that he could be strong enough to take care of my mother.

Why would he think that this surgery, at the age of eighty-one, would make him stronger? And why could he not look at his son, who had had the same cancer and survived, and not learn anything from his experience?

Because he was so afraid to change his normal. He clung to whatever therapy he thought would give him more time to live his sedentary life. To eat fatty meat three times a day, to sip brandy all day long, to never drink a glass of water. I pleaded with him to give his poor, tired body a chance, to eat a little better, to drink alcohol a bit less, to drink water to hydrate himself and cleanse his bladder and give himself a break. He would not listen, he would not change his normal, and he insisted on the surgery. Because in his mind the surgery meant he could go back to the way things were, the way that got him cancer in the first place.

The family was in horror at the prospect of the surgery. How could we keep him from fulfilling this nightmarish dream of his? Did he really think that after such a radical surgery at his age that he could go on and take care of our mother? Finally in desperation I resorted to the only thing I knew he would listen to, the only thing that could puncture the clouds in his mind. I sent him a poem from Dylan Thomas that he loved, altered with a flourish to address him more directly:

Dad,
Old age is where you find yourself. Rage against the dying
of the light. Find shelter in not knowing, find comfort in the
cold, infinite universe.
    Don't rage against oneself. Wise men know their end is

*near, but still they want to live until the last moment, whole
and complete.*

*Good men know that their deeds mean nothing, that
their lives flicker across the stage. But still they do not go
gentle into that operating room, they do not give themselves
up to the knife, they do not search for easy answers to hard
questions.*

*Wild men have learned too late how much they love life.
As they feel it slipping out of their bones they grieve life's
passing, but still they do not go gentle into that good night.*

*Grave men, facing death, can finally see the light. They
can face the truth and understand. Though they know the
end is near they still rage against the dying of the light.*

*And so you, my father, must now face your worst fears.
Out of control, out of hope, left only with love and memories.
But that is enough. It has always been enough.*

*Rage against the dying of the light, do not go gentle into
that good night.*

Your son,
Mike

With this letter I finally convinced him to take a gentler course
with his body and his cancer treatment. But still he did not do any
of the little things that could make him feel better, that could have
extended his life, that could have mitigated the cruel progress of
his disease. He was treated with chemo and could not tolerate it.
He was treated with radiation, but they irradiated his bowels so
that he died in a humiliating state of constant incontinence. I'm

grateful, though, that at least he died physically intact and with some dignity.

Through the insights of Marilu, I could see that I needed to change my normal, but it was hard to make changes. Changing normal is a very elemental exercise: it goes to the heart of who you are and what you do. The changes I had to make were deep; not only did I need to change my actions, but also who I was. The chemicals were in my body, and I could stop consuming them and gradually detox them back out. But to treat my stress, the common denominator of all my ailments, I needed to change the way I interacted with the world, the way I dealt with people. I had to change my normal.

The patient who is treated and then sent home to resume their sedentary, toxic lifestyle, like my father, is being given a death sentence. There is no sympathy from the doctor; he has moved on to his next patient. Sooner or later the cancer will come back, with even more virulence. The doctor will assure the family that there was nothing they could have done, nothing more that he could have done. The cancer came from somewhere, but no one will ever know from where. The patient will have learned the costs and limitations of his treatment, but no one will ever hear his story, his doubts, his regrets. No good will come of his brave sacrifice. All in defense of a *normal* lifestyle that is so often created by the greed of fast-food companies, big medicine, chemical plants, and pharmaceutical companies.

I had the strength to change my normal because I had changed fundamentally with the entry of Marilu into my life. My love for her had turned everything upside down. So when I was diagnosed I knew that I had something to live for and every incentive to keep my body whole. Her love for me, her instincts and intuition helped to save me. From the moment of our first date in March, two months before my diagnosis, my normal changed. I went from searching for love to searching for a way to extend my life and my health so that I could love and continue to be loved. With each change and improvement in my health, my path was reinforced. And so we hope it can be for all who read this book.

Fall 2012
Marilu

Sam Simon and I had worked together during the *Taxi* years and had even double-dated several times when I was dating his writing partner, Ken Estin, and Sam was dating soap opera producer Shelly Curtis. He and I hadn't really stayed in contact over the years, save for running into each other occasionally, until one day in September 2012, when I saw something he retweeted from Tony Danza's Twitter account and instantly started following Sam. He, in turn, followed me, and the rekindling of a friendship took place, which proves the power of social media and Twitter—with its ticker tape/Kleenex approach—in particular.

Sam and I had a lot in common, including our love of animals and extolling the virtues of all things vegetarian and vegan. Long before I had a radio show featuring celebrities and health, Sam was hosting animal lovers and activists like Ari Solomon and Pamela Anderson. By September 28, 2012, I was booked on Sam's weekly show to talk about my thirty-four-year health journey and our crazy *Taxi* past.

It was great catching up, and Sam was full of energy, as always, even though he kept explaining that he wasn't feeling his best. Less than two months later, Sam wrote and told me he had stage 4 cancer and his doctors told him it was incurable and that he had only a few months to live. I wrote and told him to call me ASAP, that I had lots of questions and would definitely connect him with the right people. When we spoke he sounded defeated and hopeless, and I said reassuringly, "You haven't talked to me yet. I'm the Doctor Concierge. Don't give up. There's no such thing as incurable until you've seen some of the people who helped Michael!"

By this time, Michael had been in remission for nine years. He remained steadfast in maintaining his protocol and had never gone back to his old normal. He'd been taking his thirty-plus tablets and capsules a day, daily exercise, hydration and rebounding, thrice-weekly infrared saunas, vegan diet, etc. When people hear what he does every day to maintain his cancer-free life, they often say, "That sounds hard." What I always tell them in reply is, "Being healthy is hard. Being unhealthy is hard. Maintaining your health is hard. Pick your hard."

I called Dr. Khalsa for Sam and arranged for the two of them to meet. Dr. Khalsa only works with patients who are serious about their health and, after talking to Sam, agreed to work with him. Sam continued to go through chemo and other medical procedures, but supplemented what his doctors were doing with Dr. Khalsa's vitamin, supplement, and food recommendations. When Sam was on my radio show in November 2014, two years after he thought he would no longer be with us, he credited Dr. Khalsa and my connecting them for giving him the extra years of life, during which time he was able to donate most of his money to improving and saving the lives of animals everywhere. He even recounted a story where he had been feeling horrible and called his oncologist, who told him to come in the following Monday. But he knew something was radically wrong and went to see Khalsa, who took one look at Sam and knew he was in sepsis and needed to be admitted to Cedars-Sinai Hospital immediately. His colon cancer doctor had perforated Sam's colon during the most recent procedure, and the poisons were about to kill him had Khalsa not insisted he be admitted.

Sam did pass away on March 8, 2015, just shy of his sixtieth birthday. I have often wondered what would have happened had he not started down the surgery and chemo road before he called me. We will never know.

The "What If?" Scenario

Michael

What if I had never contacted Marilu in February 2003? What if I had continued on my way, making marginal changes in my lifestyle with no rhyme or reason to those changes? What would have happened if I had been diagnosed by my urologist in May of that year with simple early-stage bladder cancer? And then not gotten a second opinion? And never changed my normal? What then?

My story might have gone like this:

I was diagnosed with bladder cancer in May 2003. Finally, after two years with blood in my urine, I was diagnosed properly! My doctor told me that it was a simple type of bladder cancer, that he had removed the cancer by resection, and all that I needed was a follow-up visit in September, and then he sent me home.

I was relieved by what the doctor told me, but anxious about what it all meant. The doctor had told me not to worry, to go about my life as if nothing had happened. But could I really do that? How could that be the right thing to do? The cancer had to come from somewhere! Where could I go for help?

I sought out information on the Internet and found out my treatment was the standard. There did exist an immunotherapy treatment called BCG, which could treat the tumors, but this was indicated for patients with a more advanced-stage bladder cancer, which I did not seem to have. And so I waited through the summer and was relieved that the blood in my urine had ceased. I felt fine, and as time went on my confidence increased.

Finally, the time came for my follow-up exam. I was very nervous as I drove to the clinic. My doctor told me not to worry and prepared me for surgery. I went to sleep with the anesthetic and woke up groggy and confused. This time the doctor did not come to my bedside, but instead I was released from the clinic and was told to come back for a meeting with the doctor the following week.

This wait was interminable. I thought my doctor had told me not to worry, but now here I was worrying about information that my doctor had and was holding from me! And I wondered why, if my cancer had been found at an early stage as he told me in May, did I now need to wait so long for an update on my condition? But somehow I waited through that week. When I finally got in to see the doctor, he told me that he had to wait to see me until the results of the biopsies were in. And, as it turned out, the results were not good, and the news he had to give me was not what he had expected. The cancer I had was far more advanced than he had thought back in May, though it might be that the cancer I had was so aggressive that it had moved past an early stage to an advanced stage in the short span of four months. In addition to the papillary-type tumors I also had a more aggressive tumor known as CIS, carcinoma in situ.

My head began to spin. Why had he made me wait so long for a follow-up? What could I have been doing in the meantime? And what was this CIS? And how was it to be treated?

The doctor then told me that the standard treatment for my type of bladder cancer was BCG, a special form of bovine tuberculosis injected into the bladder through a catheter. Although this treatment had been shown to be effective, it was not always, and many patients could not tolerate it. The alternative, more and more common these days, was to resect the bladder with a cystectomy, which is the surgical removal of the bladder and would also cost me my prostate gland. The downside to this procedure was that I would lose sexual function and would urinate in a bag the rest of my life, but hey, at least the cancer would be gone!

This was more information than I was ready to receive and process! A noxious chemical injected into my bladder with a low chance of success, or the removal of my bladder and prostate? What a terrible, horrific choice! But I immediately decided to go for the BCG as I did not want to lose any of my organs, no matter what.

I asked the doctor if there was anything I could be doing to help cure me of the cancer and to help me withstand the BCG treatments. "There is nothing you can do nor anything that you should do," the doctor said. "Some people believe that taking vitamins and changing the diet help, but this has never been proven." He even said that sometimes what people do to help themselves, like going on a vegan diet, actually makes things worse! The best thing I could do was to prepare my family for a difficult ordeal, but one that I could go through and have a reasonable chance to survive. And if the BCG failed, then there was always the option of surgery, though by then the cancer could have spread more widely in my body. The choice was mine.

His answer frustrated me, because I wanted to do something to help myself. Leaving it all to the doctor made me feel helpless and out of control. But his words of caution also had the ring of truth. Maybe I should not be stirring things up now, but wait until after my treatment to look at alternative ways of living. This doubt caused me to stop my search for other cures. I would trust my doctor and do as he said, he must know best.

The day finally arrived for my first BCG treatment. In the meantime I had more incidents of blood in my urine, but not as bad as before my first surgery. I went to the clinic and was checked in. I put on my gown open to the front and waited in the procedure room. The doctor and his assistant came in and had me take off my underwear and sit on the examination chair. They rubbed an ointment on my penis and testicles and then clipped a metal fastener onto my penis. The ointment was a local anesthetic and it did help. But I was nervous and was gripping the arms of the chair. They brought out a long catheter and pushed it into the head of my penis, with me squirming as they pushed it in. Finally they stopped and attached the bottle of solution to the tube and drained it into my bladder, then removed the tube and wiped the ointment off me.

I was told that I could get up and leave, but to keep the solution in my bladder for two hours. I had read on the Internet that I was supposed to lie down those two hours and roll around in different positions so that the BCG would bathe my entire bladder. When I told him that is what I wanted to do he shrugged and let me stay in the room for the two hours. As I was leaving I asked for instructions and all they said was that I might feel flulike symptoms for the next twenty-four to forty-eight hours, and to take Uribel to relieve the burning when I urinated.

Needless to say, it was not that simple. After three horrible urinations, the flulike symptoms began and those, along with the extremely painful urination, went on for two days. I felt a constant urge to pee but had very little urine to get out. I found myself drinking large amounts of water to flush out the poison, which did help. As I finally began to recover on the third day I realized with alarm that I was facing another treatment in just four days!

And so it went for five more treatments. Each time the pain of urination, the flulike symptoms, the dread of the next appointment. But I kept reminding myself that this was what I was doing to preserve my organs, to save my bladder and prostate.

Four weeks after my sixth treatment it was time to be checked by the doctor. He performed a cystoscopy, and I could tell through the haze of my anxiety that he did not like what he saw. My bladder had tolerated the BCG well enough, he said, but it had not had any effect on the tumors. It was like I had had no treatment at all.

Discouraged after the cystoscopy, I dressed and then waited to see the doctor. The cancer was growing inside me and now the only way to address the problem was to remove my bladder and prostate! I was scared and resented the fact that this was happening to me. But what could I do but go in and face the music? The doctor told me that this was a serious setback, that now surgery was definitely called for. I asked him if I could go through another round of BCG treatments, but he stood up and said to me, "You have an advanced-stage bladder cancer that is not responding to treatment. If the tumors are not removed they will spread and you could die.

Do you understand?" I nodded that I did understand, and we began to discuss the particulars of the surgery.

The surgery involved the removal of the prostate and then the bladder. A portion of my lower intestine would be used to create a neobladder. For this reason I would be able to urinate normally, rather than having the urine collect in a bag. Also, a tube would be attached to my penis; when I wanted to have sex I could inflate my penis by pumping a rubber ball attached to the tube. Again overwhelmed by information, I just shut down as he droned on. *I am screwed*, I kept thinking. *I want to die. I can't handle this.* But I made my appointment and left the office thinking about how I would deal with this monstrous problem.

Soon thereafter I had the surgery and spent months recovering. There were complications with the neobladder, and I had very little use for the penis pump. I could not exercise properly and soon I regretted having the surgery. The alternative therapies I researched were really for those who had turned down the surgery. Postsurgery, my options were much more limited. I seemed to age very quickly and a year later I felt very old indeed.

A couple of years after the surgery I got sick and began to cough up blood. Though my doctor downplayed the seriousness of this, he did request a CT scan of my chest, which, to his surprise, revealed an advanced-stage lung cancer. At first it was thought that this was metastasized bladder cancer in my lung, but it was in fact a totally separate cancer. By this time I was weak from the illness and the general malaise I felt after losing my bladder and prostate. I began to lose weight as the doctors considered my options with the lung cancer. I was treated with surgery to remove the tumor, and then chemo and radiation. I died six months later, some three years after my surgery for bladder cancer, at the age of fifty-four.

But as related in this book, my life did not go this way, though it very well could have. Because I was not alone when I was diagnosed, I found another way, one that involved taking responsibility for my health and doing what I could to change my normal and save myself. Marilu and some great doctors showed me the way out of a downward spiral, and for this I will be forever grateful.

Bibliography

Babin, Roni Caryn. "Trial of Chelation Therapy Shows Benefits, but Doubts Persist." *New York Times*, April 15, 2013. Accessed August 2, 2015. http://well.blogs.nytimes.com/2013/04/15/trial-of-chelation-therapy-shows-benefits-but-doubts-persist/?_r=0.

Bauer, Brent A., MD. "What Is an Infrared Sauna? Does It Have Health Benefits?" Mayo Clinic, June 9, 2014. Accessed June 17, 2015. http://www.mayoclinic.org/healthy-lifestyle/consumer-health/expert-answers/infrared-sauna/faq-20057954.

Beck, Melinda. "Some Cancer Experts See 'Overdiagnosis,' Question Emphasis on Early Detection." *Wall Street Journal*, September 14, 2014. Accessed October 16, 2015. http://www.wsj.com/articles/some-cancer-experts-see-overdiagnosis-and-question-emphasis-on-early-detection-1410724838.

"Bladder Cancer." Wayne State University. Accessed November 5, 2015. http://urology.med.wayne.edu/bladder.php.

"Bronchiolitis Obliterans Organizing Pneumonia." *Wikipedia*. Accessed July 7, 2015. https://en.wikipedia.org/wiki/Bronchiolitis_obliterans_organizing_pneumonia.

"Cancer Cannot Survive in an Oxygenated Alkaline Environment." Cancer Compass, 2015. Accessed October 30, 2015. http://cancercompass alternateroute.com/cancer-5/cancer-cannot-survive-in-an-oxygenated -alkaline-environment/.

Chancelor, Michael B., MD; William D. Steers, MD; and Keith N. Van Arsdalen, MD. "Cystoscopy and Ureteroscopy." National Institute of Diabetes and Digestive and Kidney Diseases. Accessed June 18, 2015. http://www .niddk.nih.gov/health-information/health-topics/diagnostic-tests/cystoscopy -ureteroscopy/Pages/default.aspx.

"Chemotherapy, Radiation Therapy and Immunotherapy." OncoSec, August 15, 2013. Accessed September 6, 2015. http://oncosec.com/chemo therapy-radiation-therapy-and-immunotherapy/.

"Definition of Electron Beam Computerized Tomography." MedicineNet. Accessed November 1, 2015. http://www.medicinenet.com/script/main/art .asp?articlekey=10296.

Dena. "My First Colonic." *Live, Love, Simple*, August 2, 2011. Accessed October 4, 2015. http://livelovesimple.com/first-colonic/.

Dolin, P. J., and P. Cook-Mozaffari. "Occupation and Bladder Cancer: A Death-Certificate Study." *British Journal of Cancer*, September 1992. Accessed September 24, 2015. http://www.ncbi.nlm.nih.gov/pmc/articles /PMC1977949/.

"EBCT Heart Scan." Orange County Heart Institute and Research Center. Accessed November 1, 2015. http://ocheartinstitute.com/EBCT_HeartFull BodyScans.html.

Egger, Garry. "The Emergence of 'Lifestyle Medicine' as a Structured Approach for Management of Chronic Disease." *Medical Journal of Australia* (2009): 144–145. https://www.mja.com.au/journal/2009/190/3/emergence -lifestyle-medicine-structured-approach-management-chronic-disease.

Freinquel, Mihal. "My First Colonic: A Trip Through My Intestines." *Huffington Post*, December 6, 2012. Accessed October 4, 2015. http://www.huff ingtonpost.com/mihal-freinquel/colonics_b_2245390.html.

Geller, Robin. "What Is the Difference Between Chemotherapy and Immunotherapy?" MadSciNetwork, September 6, 2000. Accessed October 24, 2015. http://www.madsci.org/posts/archives/2000-09/968944010.Me.r.html.

Golubic, Mladen, MD, PhD. "Lifestyle Choices: Root Causes of Chronic Diseases." Cleveland Clinic, January 14, 2013. Accessed November 3, 2015. https://my.clevelandclinic.org/health/transcripts/1444_lifestyle-choices -root-causes-of-chronic-diseases.

Greenberg, M. "Cancer Mortality in Merchant Seamen." *National Center for Biotechnology Information* (1991): 321–322. http://www.ncbi.nlm.nih.gov /pubmed/1809146.

Greger, Michael, MD. "Lifestyle Medicine: Treating the Causes of Disease." Nutrition Facts, November 4, 2013. Accessed November 3, 2015. http://nutri tionfacts.org/video/lifestyle-medicine-treating-the-causes-of-disease.

Grossarth-Matichek, R.; H. Kiene; S. M. Baumgartner; and R. Ziegler. "Use of Iscador, an Extract of European Mistletoe (Viscum Album), in Cancer Treatment: Prospective Nonrandomized and Randomized Matched-Pair Studies Nested Within a Cohort Study." *National Center for Biotechnology Information* (2001): 57–66. http://www.ncbi.nlm.nih.gov /pubmed/11347286.

Grunner, A., and W. Brunner. "The Bronchial Alveolar Carcinoma as a Solitary Coin Lesion." *National Center for Biotechnology Information* (1977): 211–12. http://www.ncbi.nlm.nih.gov/pubmed/834997.

"Hydration: Why It's So Important." Family Doctor, March 2015. Accessed July 8, 2015. http://familydoctor.org/familydoctor/en/prevention-wellness /food-nutrition/nutrients/hydration-why-its-so-important.html.

"Immunotherapy/Biological Therapy." Johns Hopkins Medicine. Accessed November 2, 2015. http://www.hopkinsmedicine.org/healthlibrary/conditions /gynecological_health/immunotherapybiological_therapy_85,P00566/.

"Intravesical Therapy for Bladder Cancer." American Cancer Society, February 25, 2015. Accessed June 20, 2015. http://www.cancer.org/cancer/bladder cancer/detailedguide/bladder-cancer-treating-intravesical-therapy.

Levine, Jonathan B., DMD. "Toxic Teeth: Are Amalgam Fillings Safe?" *The Dr. Oz Show*, March 27, 2013. Accessed June 14, 2015. http://www.doctoroz .com/article/toxic-teeth-are-our-amalgam-fillings-safe.

"Lung Needle Biopsy." Medline Plus, August 25, 2014. Accessed November 16, 2015. https://www.nlm.nih.gov/medlineplus/ency/article/003860.htm.

"Lung Needle Biopsy." Heathline. Accessed November 16, 2015. http://www .healthline.com/health/lung-needle-biopsy#Definition1.

"Merchant Marines." Mesothelioma Cancer Alliance. Accessed September 24, 2015. http://www.mesothelioma.com/asbestos-exposure/occupations /merchant-marines.htm.

Morris, Alexandra. "Cancer Immunotherapy: Hot with Promise, Potential Breakthroughs." wbur's CommonHealth Reform and Reality, February 21, 2014. Accessed November 2, 2015. http://commonhealth.wbur.org/2014/02 /cancer-immunotherapy-hot-with-promise-potential-breakthroughs.

Nicholson, William J., MD; Ruth Lilis, MD; Arthur L. Frank, MD, PhD; Irving J. Selikoff, MD. "Lung Cancer Prevalence Among Shipyard Workers." *American Journal of Industrial Medicine* 1 (2007): 191–203. Accessed September 20, 2015. http://onlinelibrary.wiley.com/doi/10.1002/ajim.4700010 210/abstract.

"Non-Small Cell Lung Cancer Treatment (PDQ®)." National Cancer Institute, May 12, 2015. Accessed July 16, 2015. http://www.cancer.gov/types /lung/patient/non-small-cell-lung-treatment-pdq.

"No Two Cancers Are the Same." Cancer Research Wales. Accessed October 30, 2015. https://www.cancerresearchwales.co.uk/blog/no-two-cancers -are-the-same/.

O'Rahilly, Ronan, MD; Fabiola Müller; Stanley Carpenter, PhD; Rand Swenson, MD, PhD. "Chapter 22: The Pleurae and Lungs." In *Basic Human*

Anatomy. Accessed June 7, 2015. https://www.dartmouth.edu/~humananat omy/part_4/chapter_22.html.

"pH and Cancer: Acidic pH Levels Can Lead to Cancer." Cancer Fighting Strategies. Accessed October 15, 2015. http://www.cancerfightingstrategies .com/ph-and-cancer.html#sthash.G4WGwqaP.dpbs.

Pityn, P.; M. J. Chamberlain; M. E. King; and W. K. Morgan. "Differences in Particle Deposition Between the Two Lungs." *National Center for Biotech-nology Information* 89 (1995). Accessed August 17, 2015. http://www.ncbi.nlm .nih.gov/pubmed/7708974.

Ruddick, Mirabelle. "Colon Hydrotherapy: What You Need to Know." *Chicago Tribune*, August 14, 2013. Accessed May 17, 2015. http://www.chicago tribune.com/suburbs/chi-ugc-article-colon-hydrotherapy-what-you-need-to -know-2013-08-14-story.html.

"Same Cancer, Different Time Zone," MD Anderson Center, July 30, 2014. Accessed September 14, 2015. http://www.mdanderson.org/newsroom/news -releases/2014/same-cancer-different-time-zone.html.

Scurr, Martin. "Why MOST Doctors Like Me Would Rather DIE than Endure the Pain of Treatment We Inflict on Others for Terminal Diseases: Insider Smashes Medicine's Big Taboo." *Daily Mail*, February 14, 2012. Accessed October 16, 2015. http://www.dailymail.co.uk/health /article-2100684/Why-doctors-like-die-endure-pain-treatment-advanced -cancer.html.

Solan, Mathew. "Walking: Your Steps to Health." Harvard Health, August 1, 2009. Accessed May 14, 2015. http://www.health.harvard.edu /newsletter_article/Walking-Your-steps-to-health.

Stram, Ronald, MD, and Sarah Stacey, FNP-C. "Mistletoe Therapy." Stram Center for Integrative Medicine, December 12, 2008. Accessed July 2, 2015. http://www.stramcenter.com/services/iscador-mistletoe-treatment/.

Ubel, Peter. "How Much Are We Over-Diagnosing Cancer?" *Forbes*, May 22, 2015. Accessed November 4, 2015. http://www.forbes.com/sites

/peterubel/2015/05/22/the-question-isnt-whether-we-are-overdiagnosing
-cancer-but-how-much/.

Ulrich, Cathy. "The Benefits of Lymphatic Massage." Massage Therapy. Accessed June 24, 2015. http://www.massagetherapy.com/articles/index.php/ar
ticle_id/1050/The-Benefits-of-Lymphatic-Massage.

"Understanding Bladder Cancer." Bladder Cancer Advocacy Network. Accessed November 5, 2015. http://www.bcan.org/learn/understanding-bladder
-cancer/.

"What Is Cystoscopy?" Urology Care Foundation. Accessed June 18, 2015.
http://www.urologyhealth.org/urologic-conditions/cystoscopy.

"What Is Small Cell Lung Cancer?" American Cancer Society, September 12,
2014. Accessed July 16, 2015. http://www.cancer.org/cancer/lungcancer-small
-cell/detailedguide/small-cell-lung-cancer-what-is-small-cell-lung-cancer.

Work, Chris. "The Best Exercise for Your Immune System: Rebounding!"
Chris Beat Cancer, August 10, 2012. Accessed May 10, 2015. http://www.chris
beatcancer.com/rebounding/.

Acknowledgments

Marilu

Whenever people asked how Michael and I got together, they'd hear our story and say, "This has to be a book!" We knew we wanted to share our journey and the knowledge we gained in the process with the world, but it had to be with a team that would let us tell the story without holding back. We pitched the idea to Jen Bergstrom at Simon & Schuster who immediately said, "I love it!" Not many publishers would be so forthcoming, and that's what makes her the coolest publisher in the business (as well as the best dressed!). Thank you, Jenn! To her team at Simon & Schuster: A huge thank-you to Kate Dresser, editor extraordinaire, for her talent and vigilance, and for being the Couples Whisperer; to Becky Prager for assisting Kate in keeping this project on track; and to Jennifer Robinson with whom I had so much fun promoting *Total Memory Makeover*. I can't wait to do it again.

To Pete Sanders, publicist and friend, for always making sure I get the word out in the most effective way possible.

To Jeff Katz for his extraordinary book cover photos and patience while working with two very different subjects.

To Mel Berger from WME, the best literary agent anyone can have. Our tenth book together, and I love you more and more with each one.

To my long-standing team at Innovative Artists: Jonathan Howard, Nevin Dolcefino, Marcia Hurwitz, Steve LaManna, and Brian Davidson.

To my radio show gang, who shares with me one of my favorite experiences ever: Gina Yates, Denise McIntee, Steve Guzman, and Mondo Hernandez. I love you guys!

To the great tag team of assistants: the efficient Courtney Salmon, who started the research and handed it off to the effervescent Nicki Hirschorn, who passed it to the ever-steady Aliya Stuart, who was always on top of the bibliography and photos.

To my BFFs for their unwavering love and support: the irrepressible Cynthia Wilkerson for reading the drafts and speaking her mind; the outrageous Sharon Feldstein for her fashion, psychic, and doctor expertise; and the talented MaryAnn Hennings for her magic and makeovers throughout the years, including the fabulous photos for this and every book!

To Dr. Neal Barnard, Nelson Campbell, and Dr. T. Colin Campbell for their extraordinary knowledge and books that ride the highest wave in the tsunami of health; and to Fran Drescher, health advocate and founder of Cancer Schmancer—thank you all for the cover quotes that lend credibility to our book. And to the incomparable Dr. Soram Khalsa for his inquisitive nature and continued diagnostic genius, and for his refreshingly honest foreword to this book. Michael would not be here without you.

To Lorin Henner for your overview, insights, and humor when we needed it most, which was always. Our tenth book together made even more special this time because of your adorable children, Joe and Katherine.

And to my remarkable guys Nick and Joey Lieberman, for being the best part of life's journey, with an extra thanks to Nick for your talent as a writer, editor, and, especially, referee!

Michael

I would like to acknowledge the many people who helped me through this health journey. Many of them are mentioned in the book, especially Dr. Soram Khalsa, Dr. Sharron Mee, Dr. Joel Wachtel, Dr. Keith Block, Dr. Robert McKenna, and Dr. Donald Lamm (through his research). All of these fine doctors were aided by so many fine nurses and staff who became friends during the journey. Thanks to the staff at Clear Way to Health, especially Laura Weeks and Talya, who quickly became friends and mentors.

Marilu's family welcomed me and put up with a lot that first year! Nicky and Joey Lieberman, of course, and the rest of the family—Greg Siegel and Liz Carney and their son, Jackson, born the day after that first reunion dinner with Marilu; Suzy Carney and Charlotte; Tom Alderman and Melody Henner; Tommy Henner; Christal Henner and her boys, Christopher and William; and JoAnn Carney and the man himself, William Drake. Being accepted by them so readily made my life's transition much easier.

My colleagues at BrownTrout Publishers were very supportive.

Thanks to Jack and Gail Straw, Michael Reif, Bob and Meg John-son, Samanta Anguiano, David and Julie Taff, Andrew Anderson, Sharon Levine, and so many more. My partner and friend Marc Winkelman and his wife, Suzanne, and their children Ellie, Alex, and Jacob; I am so thankful to be a part of their life. Thanks to my buddy and mentor Joe Angard and his wife, Susan; Joe's positive spirit has kept me going now for so many years. And a special ac-knowledgment to Tom Bove, with whom I have shared many chal-lenges and who himself saw the power of changing normal a few years after my illness.

My mother and father, LaRae and Bill, were always there for me, even if I could not see it at times. As were my sister, Julie, and her husband, Jon Larsen; my twin brother, Marc, and his wife, Wendo-ver, and their son, Marc; Rob Brown and his son Max and ex-wife Jeanine. My dear aunt Margaret, who passed away from cancer as I was recovering, a great loss to me and her dear family. So many kind cousins from Utah and Idaho who have stayed close to me through the years and keep me grounded and in touch with my roots. I would especially like to thank and acknowledge my children: Carine and Andy and their children Malia and Maya Santiago; Cassia and Joe Morris and her children Victoria and Lucas Robertson; and to my son, Michael. They have been with me through the bad times and the good, and I am thankful for them every day.

Finally I would like to acknowledge all those people who have fought the good fight against cancer. Those who have grown to love their bodies even more as they confront this awful disease. Those who refuse to accept easy answers and try to understand how they can help themselves to find a cure that works for them. Lonesome warriors who have led the way, and through their courage helped me to find my way back to health and a positive future.